Buddha Belly

Maryann,

Congrats on your 2018 journey.

Betty Phelps

Buddha Belly

A Mind-Body-Soul Approach to Health Starting with Your Gut

BRITTNEY L PRENDERGAST CHC

ISBN: 1539543234
ISBN 13: 9781539543237

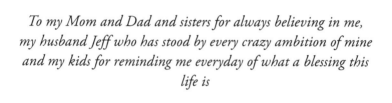

*To my Mom and Dad and sisters for always believing in me,
my husband Jeff who has stood by every crazy ambition of mine
and my kids for reminding me everyday of what a blessing this
life is*

Table of Contents

Introduction

*"Once you make a decision, the universe
conspires to make it happen"*

RALPH W. EMERSON

*E*very great change requires a decision. I love Emerson and
his life philosophies for a lot of reasons. He was an emotionally intuitive, deep thinker and I feel that he understood
the necessary balance of mind, body and soul while truly
valuing the intangible. I have come to learn that true health
is multi-faceted and can only be achieved when all aspects,
mental, emotional, physical and spiritual, come into alignment. If we wish to transform our bodies and our lives, we
have to nurture all aspects of ourselves.

I started this book at the beginning of my health and life
coaching career/journey because I wanted to put on paper for
the world everything that I had learned from my experiences

up until and through this place in my own life. For the previous decade I have considered myself a "health nut". Not because I ate perfectly or even ideally but because I sucked up all the knowledge I could about nutrition, disease, prevention, stress and anything "healthy" that I could get my hands on! This consists of over one hundred books and tons of Internet reading, along with my own ever evolving health choices. I've experimented with different foods, diets and lifestyles as well as observing the health and quality of life in those around me.

Growing up I was very overweight. I can still remember what it felt like to be made fun of and the feeling of being ashamed through the better part of my childhood. I developed an emotional attachment to food at an early age which later morphed into a dieting obsession and a constant state of inadequacy. As I got older I restricted calories and ate minimal amounts of nutrient-poor foods in an effort to lose pounds while counting every calorie burned on cardio equipment.

These naive practices resulted in weight loss but also muscle and nutrient loss and it did nothing for the other demons that plagued me: the severe anxiety and patchy depression that I experienced for as long as I can remember. Although I have never been "skinny", I maintained a healthy weight for most of my adult years. Even still, I have spent the better part of every day for the majority of my life relentlessly thinking about food and judging my own physical form.

In my early 20's I got married and focused every moment of free time I had to reading about health and working out. I became a vegetarian and over that 5 year period of time, I found myself unable to get pregnant. When I finally did, I miscarried my desired baby. Knowing what I know now, this was a big sign that my hormones were not in alignment and my stress and attempt to be "healthy" had damaged my adrenals, but I did not give that intuition enough attention. Shortly after that I conceived my first angel baby boy.

When my son was one and a half I went through a painful divorce. In the few years following my divorce I remarried and soon after, experienced another miscarriage. At that point I started looking into the hormonal implications of the lifestyle I was following and found it to be much less "healthy" then I had thought. A few months after the second miscarriage, life brought a whirlwind of unexpected, debilitating family occurrences at which point, my personal health was the last thing on my mind. However, like the Phoenix rises from the ashes, so did I and my family. But, I knew that along with the long road of emotional healing, my body needed healing too; not just physical healing from stress and trauma, but true healing in all areas of my health.

During the unexpected conception of my second healthy boy, my husband and I made the decision to give up my retail business which allowed me to spend time nurturing myself and my family while diving deeper into my new found understanding of wellness. This decision led me to a new life fulfilling "career" with passion and clarity. I got my certification in holistic health and life coaching and use this alongside my previous self-education and experience to fuel my knowledge and drive. I have come to understand the immense role of the immune system and its origin in the gut. I feel our gut health is the key to overcoming so many issues and ailments.

You may wonder why this book is titled "Buddha Belly". It isn't a pun on weight and honestly, it's not because I am a Buddhist, but because the Buddhist often emulate this multi-dimensional form of health and have the documented longevity and quality of life to show for it. As a health and life coach I don't just focus on the physical body. I have a passion to help people strengthen their physical health while nurturing their mind and listening to their soul. True transformation comes from the inside out, through life giving foods, self-love, peace and personal understanding of who you truly are. This book is to be used right where you are today, because now is the moment you've chosen to change your future.

Once a person decides what they desire and gives themselves permission to live it and be it, it will be. I have a healthier mind, body and soul now, more than any other time in my life because I gave myself permission to live my intention and made the decision that now it will be so. My passion doesn't come from money or personal gratification but from an honest desire to empower everyone toward their life's purpose through optimum health, while invoking confidence in each of them to know that they are powerful, strong and beautiful.

Although it may be a long road toward the outcome, every step along the path will motivate and nurture you to a better place than the step before. Decide what it is you want, make your decision and may this book be your first step.

One

What brings you here?

Life is about constantly evolving, meaning that everything is possible. One of my favorite motivational speakers, Anthony Robbins, put it best; "The only impossible journey is the one you never take." Where do you stand today and what has brought you here? Is it illness, weight problems, anxiety, depression, infertility, struggles with self-esteem, digestive distress or a combination of these? What is holding you back from living vibrantly in this life? This book's main focus is balancing the gut and empowering the body to achieve its optimal physical state. However, the balancing of life and who we are as people is a crucial component in achieving true transformation.

Is your desire to improve your physical body, mind-body or emotional self? Hopefully you will see a healthy evolution in all of these areas by the end of this process. There are many "diets" out there, but the intent behind this book is aimed at achieving a healthy state of being, using the most crucial tool to physical health, the GUT, while nurturing your mind and body into the best version of itself. Diet related issues are rarely just a lack of knowledge about what to eat. The psychology behind eating behaviors is quite complex and through my personal experience, it requires a different approach.

When I was half way through my certification as a holistic health and life coach, I had the pleasure of meeting an interesting woman who had written many diet books. After engaging with her about her accomplishments I then told her about the direction I was headed with my program. After asking about the specific course that I was taking, her first response was "Health <u>and</u> life coaching? What an odd combination. I've never heard of that before". My program was the only one that offered both a health and life coaching certification, but I found her remark enlightening. Bless her heart, here was a woman with years of experience in holistic health and writing who had some excellent dietary knowledge, yet appeared to have little understanding of what I call the "Mind and Soul" part of health. Because of the interconnection between life and health, I couldn't understand why these two areas of coaching hadn't been married earlier!

To understand health from a natural, holistic perspective it is important to understand that the body is an intricately designed machine. In order to function well, it must achieve synchronicity with not only it's physical self, but it's mental, emotional and spiritual self. This is why it is crucial to listen to the body's communication. Symptoms such as insomnia, fatigue, depression, anxiety, infertility, excess weight, irregular elimination, skin problems, food allergies and headaches are all examples of the body sending you signals that something more complex is out of whack. Unfortunately, in our modern age, we are taught to seek medication to "band-aid "the signal, instead of following it to the source. Think of these bodily cues like a smoke alarm. What good would it do for us to just remove the batteries every time the smoke alarm went off? Sure, it would stifle that high pitch annoyance, meanwhile allowing a fire to potentially consume our home and loved ones. Not worth it. Your body works just like the fire alarm, alerting you of danger before it's too late. I personally don't believe any symptoms or suffering happens without a deeper root cause, worthy of investigation.

The great thing about our magnificent bodies is that they are resilient and want to heal. Even some of the most far-gone bodies are in a constant state of repair. What we need to do is let the body do its job by nourishing it properly, nurturing it and loving it through the process. As overwhelming as the journey may feel, especially if you are suffering from multiple symptoms, keep in mind that the important part is that you start somewhere. The understanding and theories about where many of these symptoms originate from are evolving by the day, especially within the holistic community.

Many individuals seek out diet programs and workout regimens; some healthy, some not so much, in order to heal or change their bodies to no avail. Being hungry and stressed out is no way to live and neither is counting calories. Seeing yourself critically with negative judgements and poor self-esteem is no quality of life either. Many Americans live on what I consider "prescription life support", meaning they function fine enough but are dependent on daily pharmaceuticals which come with not only negative side effects, but also the consequence of a further damaged gut lining and liver.

With the evolving information now available about the human microbiome, or "gut", we are able to understand that by balancing this area of the body we have the ability to improve or heal the entirety of symptoms in the majority of suffering individuals. So much damage has been done to the human gut with processed foods, chemicals and an all too accepted level of chronic stress. It's time to educate our society about the importance of a healthy microbiome and the severe issues brought forth by a modern lifestyle so that we can find hope in our bodies and our future. We deserve to live with less reliance on prescription drugs and we need to stop wasting moments watching life pass us by without being a thriving contribution to it. All the while learning to love ourselves throughout the process.

Whether you picked up this book due to struggles with weight, emotional distress, digestive distress, or simply out of curiosity, thank you for joining the growing number of individuals who are empowering the rest of the world to jump on board and educate themselves, refusing to accept a mediocre or poor quality of life, living in fear of cancer and disease. Listen to your body when it speaks. This will be important to remember throughout this process because it will enable you to decipher the current state of YOUR body and use the information to navigate the best approaches for YOU.

Two

IS YOUR GUT MAKING YOU STRONGER OR WEAKER?

It's not new to hear about how disease is on the rise in industrialized cultures. Type-2 Diabetes continues to be one of the number one killers and unfortunately is now effecting younger and younger generations. Fifteen years ago, finding a child or adolescent with Type-2 Diabetes was rare and now it's become prominent enough that they changed the name from "adult onset diabetes" to "type two." It is not a coincidence that this, along with Heart Disease and cancer have risen consistently with expanding waistlines, processed foods and modern lifestyle.

We don't live in the same world as our grandparents did. Moderate amounts of substances that don't even classify as food are different then occasional amounts of real butter, fat and unprocessed sugars. The "everything in moderation" rule is now providing a quick ticket to a damaged inner ecosystem; especially because the average person believes many artificial foods to be within the "healthy" category. While most people understand the correlation between poor diet, inactivity and modern disease, a new understanding of how these negative behaviors impact our microbiome and thus influence our susceptibility to disease is an emerging discovery. I personally give credit to the underground wellness community, the group of holistic practitioners, naturalists and the like who have made a mission of questioning the root causes of these conditions and how to prevent and heal them, instead of just "band- aiding" the symptom.

The role that the gut plays in disease is incredible and despite this wealth of knowledge, there is still so much more to learn. First a quick explanation of the human microbiome "gut." The body's microbiome is a partner to the genome (genes). The human microbiome is a combination of live microbial bacteria and outnumbers the amount of genes 10 to 1. Yes, we are more bacteria then we are human genes! The intestinal tract and entire gut consist of multiple types of bacteria; some good, some bad. The ideal ratio of good bacteria to bad is 85% good to 15% bad. This allows the immune strengthening bacteria to have the upper hand against disease and sickness. Not surprisingly then that the average individual eating the standard American diet has a bacterial balance of 15% good to 85% bad. This ratio sheds a lot of light on the epidemic levels of rising illness in industrialized cultures. Our good bacteria represent our "fighters." These bacteria are the ones we want to fight off all the scary stuff. If the average person is walking around with a pitiful representation of an immune system and is already overwhelmed with the "bad guys", then how are we supposed to take on foreign invaders like the flu, not to mention a larger, more debilitating illness?

People who get sick a lot most likely have an off-kilter microbiome balance. What causes a poor microbiome ratio? Many things, but one being antibiotics. The word anti biotic literally means "against life" and used for the purpose of killing bacteria. Unfortunately, antibiotics aren't discriminatory and dissipate anything in their path, including our "fighters." Don't get me wrong, as natural as I am, the discovery of antibiotics has saved countless lives and are a blessing in our modern world. With that said, I personally don't let them near myself or my children unless it's an obvious need or other natural methods have not worked. In the five years of my oldest son's life, he's been on antibiotics once for an ear infection as a compromise with my ex-husband. I didn't eat clean while pregnant, birth un-medicated and breastfeed for nothing! Those hard-earned microbes are precious and as a mother I am conscious about wiping them away with antibiotics, especially for what was possibly a viral infection, where antibiotics are useless anyway. This is why self-education is so important, especially for a parent. The human body was designed to do incredible things. For this reason, educate yourself and be discriminatory as to what you allow in the bodies of you and yours.

Food or "Food"

Another microbial destroyer is obviously a modern diet of processed, highly chemical laden "food." Although processed foods existed throughout the 20th century, it wasn't until the 1950's that they started consuming the American household (no pun intended). The influx of fast food restaurants and highly processed frozen cuisine provided easy meals for the average busy parent and with the depression era over, families could afford these modern meals instead of relying heavily on plant based garden foods like beans, rice and veggies. Products were advertised as "fortified" meaning they contained synthetic vitamins, which manipulated the public into believing that these foods could qualify as a healthy addition to their children's diets.

While digging through some old pictures and keepsakes, my mother recently came across a written recommendation from her childhood pediatrician, advising my grandmother to start adding Jell-O to my infant mother's diet. Aside from the benefits of gelatin which you can obtain from much healthier sources, there is absolutely no reason to feed an infant or any child for that matter, processed, sugar laden, artificially colored, and full of preservatives, Jell-O.

"Real, healthy food doesn't come with a food label." The additives and ingredients in processed foods have a detrimental effect on the human gut. In a recent article by Dr. Mercola, he talks about the difference between types of sugar and inflammation, which is present in chronic diseases such as diabetes, heart disease and stroke. Simple sugars increase inflammation markers in the blood, whereas the non-starchy, complex carbohydrate sugars found in fruits and vegetables actually reduce these markers.

Not only do processed foods contain additives and unhealthy types of sugars, but they are often full of unhealthy fats such as hydrogenated oils. These oils are basically a vegetable oil injected with hydrogen molecules, allowing it to sit solid at room temperatures. This same process also allows it to sit solid in the walls of our arteries, further exacerbating a chronic state of inflammation. With so much junk floating around in convenience foods and causing destruction to our beloved microbiome, we must keep in mind the importance of choosing foods which don't have labels.

Our modern lifestyle is playing a major part in worsening gut health. The high stress, constant "go, go, go" mentality and financial pressures have caused a massive cortisol imbalance contributing to leaky gut which is why I have devoted an entire chapter in this book about stress and gut health. Along with the use of antibacterial soaps, chemical cleaners and body care, pasteurized animal products, pesticide laden foods and pharmaceuticals, the human gut is losing the war against disease. The war it was created to fight for us and our well-being. Antibacterial soaps do just what they promise; kill bacteria, all bacteria, including the good. Pasteurization of raw milk is another way we have stripped otherwise healthy products of their benefits. Pasteurization has mutilated the beneficial enzymes in dairy leaving it with very little health benefits, especially considering the antibiotics and hormones also present.

We are killing our microbiome with painkillers and pesticides

Painkillers and pharmaceuticals have become all too easy. Sometimes it is necessary to take a painkiller, but we've gotten too used to relying on them for every ache and pain. Those headaches and pains are usually the body communicating to us. Not only are we using a pill to "shut off the alarm," but we are also causing more depletion of our bacterial reserves. Recent studies have shown that 2 weeks on a NSAID or non-steroidal anti-inflammatory drugs (painkillers) has a 75% chance of causing intestinal permeability or leaky gut. In addition to contributing to leaky gut, painkillers are hard on the liver. Your liver is your body's filtration system. Your gut and your liver go hand in hand and both need to be functioning smoothly for optimal health to occur. Herbal remedies and holistic options have been around for years and have proven quite effective in pain elimination and healing while being a less destructive option for your liver and your gut.

The massive negative implications of non-organic foods sprayed with chemical pesticides are something that can no longer be ignored. Non-organic foods are treated with insecticides and pesticides designed to keep infestation off of crops and bugs away from our food. Unfortunately, anything designed to kill a bug will wipe out our positive bacteria and has no place in our food. Along with hybridized, genetically modified foods, the tomato of yesterday hardly resembles the tomato of today, and your body knows the difference.

We get it from our momma!

We get our first dose of bacteria when passing through the birth canal of our mothers. Her bacterial flora is the first dose of immune system we are introduced to. Needless to say, if mom is lacking in this area baby will likely get sub-par bacteria. The baby will get significantly less if birthed through C-section. Dr. David Williams enlightened his readers with the stats of declining microbial bacteria in proceeding generations, basically showing that our poor diets have led to a poor bacterial gut balance that we are passing on to our children, who pass on even less to their children and so on. All the while chronic disease keeps climbing. For those who know the importance of exposure to maternal bacterial flora, I have heard documented cases of couples, who after an unplanned C-section, swabbed the newborns ears, mouth and body with bacteria from the mother. I think this is an amazingly intelligent idea and with luck, this practice will hopefully find its way into mainstream medicine.

Starting here

This book is a massive start to improving your immune system and through the process you will experience the shedding of pounds as well as unwanted symptoms. The gut is being referred to as "the second brain." Michael Gershon, author of "The second brain" and chairman of the Department of Anatomy and Cell Biology at New York–Presbyterian Hospital/Columbia University Medical Center, is an expert in the nascent field of neurogastroenterology. He explains that the second brain has a multitude of neurons which enable us to "feel" our insides. These neurons allow the intestines to act separately of the brain such as the involuntary contracting involved in digesting and moving waste and food. It is also responsible for the majority of the serotonin produced in the body.

When the body is nourished and the gut is functioning well, it will be obvious in multiple aspects of a person, from physical improvement to mental and emotional health. Hopefully you now have enough understanding of the human microbiome to appreciate all the emerging information surrounding it and feel motivated to strengthen your own inner ecosystem. The reason so many individuals improve their diet and lifestyle but still don't see the level of improvement they are striving for in their symptoms may be because they haven't healed the root of the problem; the quality of the gut. It's time to embrace "germs" in the right way and use them to protect ourselves from illness and disease so we can get to fully living.

Three

LEAKY GUT

What is "Leaky Gut"? Leaky gut is a term used to describe intestinal hyper-permeability and the range of issues associated with it. When the gut lining becomes permeable it basically becomes filled with holes much larger and out of control then nature intended. A healthy digestive lining is like a fine netting, letting chosen nutrients through and into the body while keeping foreign bodies inside the digestive tract where they can be eliminated properly. When this "net" is damaged, the holes become greater thus allowing objects into the blood stream that the body wasn't made to take on. The presence of these foreign bodies in the blood first over tax the liver, causing it to filter substances that should have been filtered in the gut. Because the liver can't possibly keep up with this level of filtration, the floating debris now awakens the body's immune system to prepare for a full blown "attack."

This attack is very taxing on the immune system. When intestinal permeability is left untreated, only to further worsen, the bodies constant state of fight leads to chronic inflammation. Inflammation occurs when the body sends white blood cells into its tissues, inflaming them in order to protect itself from damage done by foreign substances. This is a protective action, however, if constant debris such as food particles caused by leaky gut are entering the blood, constant inflammation will occur. Think of this as having a fever every day of your life. Inflammation is an immune response and has been found to be present in most if not all chronic diseases such as diabetes, cancer, heart disease, depression and digestive related issues like IBS. With the presence of inflammation consistent with so many chronic diseases, healing a leaky gut not only has the power to reduce inflammation but prevent or reverse these epidemic levels of disease.

"Leaky gut" has been a controversial topic between holistic practitioners and the typical medical community:

["Leaky gut syndrome is a hypothetical, medically unrecognized condition which some alternative health practitioners claim is the cause of a wide range of serious chronic diseases, including diabetes, lupus, and multiple sclerosis. Proponents claim that poor diet, parasites, infection, or medications cause damage to the intestinal wall or lining, permitting toxins, microbes, undigested food, or other substances to leak through. According to the hypothesis, this "leakage" prompts the body to initiate an immune reaction that, in turn, leads to chronic diseases such as those mentioned. [1]

The "leaky gut" hypothesis is vague and largely unproven, and the scientific community continues to debate whether "leaky gut syndrome" exists at all. There is no credible evidence that any chronic diseases are caused by a "leaky" gut, nor that any remedies marketed for its treatment bring the benefits they claim. "Wikipedia"

"Leaky gut syndrome" is said to have symptoms including bloating, gas, cramps, food sensitivities, and aches and pains. But it's something of a medical mystery. "From an MD's standpoint, it's a very gray area," says gastroenterologist Donald Kirby, MD, director of the Center for Human Nutrition at the Cleveland Clinic. "Physicians don't know enough about the gut, which is our biggest immune system organ."

"Leaky gut syndrome" isn't a diagnosis taught in medical school. Instead, "leaky gut really means you've got a diagnosis that still needs to be made," Kirby says. "You hope that your doctor is a good-enough Sherlock Holmes, but sometimes it is very hard to make a diagnosis." ~Web MD]

As you can see, the topic is touchy for some. It often appears to be a "which came first the chicken or the egg?" situation. Is Leaky Gut really illusive and unspecific, distracting us from an acute issue? Or is Leaky Gut a very real side effect of poor diet and lifestyle, which sets into motion all following disease?

Many highly respected and highly educated medical doctors support the ladder and fully believe the Leaky Gut "theory." Dr. Josh Axe has done immense work on this topic, after watching his mother's cancer return shortly after her conventional medical treatments of chemo and radiation. A physician himself, Dr. Axe talks about taking time off to spend with his mother upon the return of her cancer, to "Do something more natural." He then had her follow a strict gut healing plan and her oncologist was shocked to watch her tumor shrink consistently until she no longer had a mass. She now lives vibrant and free of cancer.

Sometimes it takes disease in ourselves or those close to us, to find the motivation to dig deeper to find the root of our suffering. Especially for those already indoctrinated in the current state of medicinal practice. In his book, "Clean Gut", Dr. Alejandro Junger describes his own physical issues with illness, weight and blood pressure. What was very interesting however was his emotional account of his own severe depression. He saw that conventional treatment using pharmaceuticals were not "curing" the problem, but "band-aiding" the symptoms, leading to more issues and a further need of pills and potions. He then went on a spiritual as well as physical "detox" over in India. While there he meditated daily and followed a strict, healing diet. After leaving the facility, he was 15 lbs. lighter and his depression had lifted along with his dependency on prescriptions.

Despite modern medicine's skepticism, I feel that like Junger, the many people who have transformed their bodies and their lives through healing their gut are enough to give it merit. Like Dr. Junger points out, some individuals have deeper lying issues such as parasites or heavy metals which will stand in the way of full recovery, but through the process of gut healing and functional medicine these things can be discovered.

I am not a medical doctor myself and always recommend that my clients work with a doctor (naturopath preferably) if they are suffering with severe symptoms so that deeper issues can be addressed and avoided, and the right combination of supplements and medications can be administered safely. Even then, most people should still be able to follow a gut balancing protocol without conflict.

Leaky gut is a result of living against what nature intended

What causes Leaky Gut? Sometimes it feels like the shorter explanation is, what doesn't? An abundance of real organically produced fruits and veggies, moderate amounts of wild (or as close to wild as possible) animal products along with quality sleep will NOT give you a leaky gut! Long walks in the woods, breathing fresh air and daily quiet meditation or yoga won't give it to you either. These examples are the balance nature intended for us: to be swift but not rushed, fed for nourishment not gluttony, and surrounded by companionship with a gratitude for the daily gift of life.

As discussed in chapter 2, we have come a long way from this primitive yet simple way of life. A constant deadline, rush hour traffic and an over booked schedule has left our cortisol levels (stress hormones) skyrocketing. Lack of time for quality in our relationships as well as our food has left us undernourished and disconnected. Because we have come so far from healthy balance, the thought of healing ourselves can feel overwhelming, but the key is to start somewhere. So let's start with food.

The food we eat has had major consequences on our Gut

Gluten (a protein found in wheat) is a big offender. Gluten is hard to digest for a lot of people and absolutely atrocious for others. For people with a gluten sensitivity, eating gluten causes the immune system to go into hyper-drive and actually destroy the gut lining leading to Leaky Gut. People with Celiac Disease, which is an allergy to gluten, experience horrific side effects.

Even those without Celiac however, are still largely effected by the substance due in large part to the type of gluten based products that currently exist. Today, many forms of gluten containing foods such as wheat, barley and rye are hybridized, meaning the genetic makeup is altered from its natural state. This is done to achieve pest control, climate tolerance and profitability. The result? A form of nutrient which the body is already sensitive to, now becomes unrecognizable. The immune system will now call an attack at some level. Mankind currently over consumes gluten in the form of processed foods. Along with other "frankenutrients," the

constant immune response to our foods and the foreign con-
taminants is tearing our guts apart.

Corn for instance, is a highly gut irritating food, especially because ninety percent of corn is genetically modified
and used for high fructose corn syrup (HFCS), a chemically
processed, concentrated form of sugar made from Genetically
Modified Organism (GMO) corn. This "sugar" syrup has
now taken place of most typical sugar in processed foods and
is present in everything from cereals to ketchup and bread.
The response to HFCS by the body is not the same as authen-
tic sugar. The body is intelligent and knows this substance is a
foreign chemical therefore it reacts differently. High fructose
corn syrup does not trigger the same satiation response in the
brain (the que that you've had enough). This is especially concerning because almost all soda is produced using HFCS.

In my opinion, one of the fastest ways to shut down your
pancreas and become a type two diabetic is to drink soda.
Not only is it full of "chemicalized sugar", drinking it throws
it into your system with absolutely no fiber to slow it down.
I'm not a perfectionist but as a mom and health educator, I
strongly preach against giving your children soda unless you
want to give them a fast track to a hospital bed, wreck their
gut and insure their early dependency on pharmaceuticals.

The fake stuff is no better

Artificial sweeteners such as Saccharin, Aspartame and
Sucralose are a chemical, not a food. Many countries don't
even let these products across their borders because of the

potential health consequences. These sweeteners are found in all diet sodas and "sugar free" processed foods and should be absolutely avoided. Not only can they trick the body into producing insulin it doesn't need, they easily cause sweet cravings from other sources as an attempt to stabilize low blood sugars. Along with their counterintuitive effects, they are also very dangerous. Studies have shown links between artificial sweeteners and odd tumor masses on the brain and side effects such as vision problems, seizures, MS and cancers and that's the short list. Rather than take up an entire chapter discussing the pitfalls of artificial sweeteners, I will encourage you to seek out all the information you can, if this is an area of concern for you. The documentary "Sweet Misery" is highly informative and will make you think twice before that next sugar free, latte. Just remember "sugar free" means "chemical rich."

Our food is loaded with chemicals

Chemicals and preservatives used to extend the shelf life of packaged foods are another offender causing a similar attack by the immune system. Natural, healthy foods are not only label-less, they also rot. In order to give foods excessive shelf life, packaged foods are made with preservatives. Although natural preservation methods exist such as canning and smoking, most packaged goods are preserved by using chemical substances to keep the food "shelf stable." This is why some forms of "food" look identical to the day they were manufactured after a ridiculous amount of time has passed. Having chemicals like these roaming the walls of your arteries is not only toxic, it stresses the body like a slow embalming process. Your gut is worth more than a fluffy, cream filled, chemical concoction.

A word about stress and pills

Stress plays a significant role in leaky gut (which we will get into in chapter 6) but the usage of pharmaceuticals has also wreaked havoc. Common pain killers such as Aspirin, Ibuprofen and Naproxen wear down the protective mucosal lining of the gut. This not only leaves the guts precious "netting" more exposed and vulnerable to damage, it also irritates the gut bacteria, throwing it off balance. As addressed in chapter 2, the presence of positive gut bacteria is of utmost importance. When we weaken these pro-lifers, we allow an overgrowth of negative bacteria. The gut microbes respond to painkillers differently. A study in the Pharmaceutical Journal explained that gut microbes react to painkillers and prescriptions in a multitude of ways such as producing toxic bi-products, activating or inactivating drugs and have the ability to alter how the drugs are metabolized by human cells. According to Ramy Aziz, a microbiologist in the faculty of Pharmacy at Cairo University, "You can give two people the same drug and they will respond differently. And it's not because of their genes but because of the difference in the microbes they carry."

Signs of leaky gut

Signs of Leaky Gut can be few or many. Because bacterial quality and quantity differ from person to person, along with the extent of permeability, symptoms can very both in manifestation and severity. A few examples include, chronic digestive problems (gas, bloating and irregular elimination), nutritional deficiencies, poor immune system (getting sick frequently), headaches, excessive fatigue, skin issues (rashes, eczema, acne), sugar and carb cravings, arthritis/joint pain, depression and associated mental challenges (Attention Deficit Disorder/Hyperactivity Disorder), autoimmune diseases (Rheumatoid Arthritis, Lupus, Celiac and Crohn's diseases), just to name a few.

When the body starts attacking itself

Autoimmune diseases are particularly frightening and on a steady incline. Autoimmune disease occurs when your immune system, which is meant to fight foreign invaders, mistakes your own healthy tissues as foreign and calls an attack. This will happen in different areas of the body depending on the type of autoimmunity. For instance, a thyroid disorder is when the immune system attacks the thyroid, rheumatoid arthritis is where the immune system attacks the lining of joints and sometimes even the eyes, skin, lungs, heart and blood vessels. As listed previously, there are many forms of autoimmune disease however the question still begs, "Why are they increasing?" You may be surprised to know that autoimmune disease effects 24 million Americans. So far 80 diseases have been classified as autoimmune and the list keeps growing. Collectively, this becomes a scary reality, especially because some of these include things like MS or Muscular Sclerosis where the immune system eats away at the protective covering surrounding the nerves, leading to painful bouts of debilitation and possibly taking years off one's life. In conventional medical treatments, we have been taught that more medication is needed to treat the symptoms of these diseases, without guidance on how to decipher and treat the root cause.

Dr. Mark Hyman is one of many who has been very outspoken about his position on Functional Medicine (a form of medical practice focusing on the root cause and working therapeutically with the patient to address the true issue). He has spoken about what he believes is needed to heal most autoimmune disorders, even the ones deemed by the medical community as "incurable." He has his patients' follow a list of dietary and lifestyle changes, including treating leaky gut and searching for underlining issues such as parasites and heavy metals. He even lists adequate sleep as an important factor toward a healthy healing process.

Although the cause of autoimmunity is still claimed to be unknown, we can assert that like many "western diseases" it has risen with our industrialized ways of life such as food, lifestyle, environment and stress. So why would it seem so impossible that perhaps we can do something about it? Not only prevent it from occurring but even lessen or completely reverse the suffering of currently diagnosed individuals. There is at least enough momentum now from the holistic community, giving us plenty of information and allowing us to make our own educated opinions about how our care will be handled and what it can look like in the long term.

Mental illness isn't just in your head

A lesser acknowledged symptom of leaky gut is mental illness. The prevalence of depression and anxiety in western cultures is heartbreaking. For those who have seen the consequences of this affliction, it can be a traumatic experience. Rather its oneself or a close friend or loved one, these types of diseases hurt and sometimes take lives. Ninety percent of serotonin (happy hormone) is made in the gut. Yet everyday more and more people are prescribed gut damaging anti-depressants and anti-anxiety medications, only to continue suffering. Now that we've discovered the brain gut connection, hope in winning the battle over mental illness is a very real truth.

Because of the prevalence of Leaky Gut and all that is believed to be associated with it, Buddha Belly focuses on this area of the physical body while connecting it to mind/body health. My personal passion is helping others recognize these connections while discovering balance and love for their own bodies. Buddha Belly will give you tools and information as well as hopefully a motivation to nurture yourself.

What to expect

At the end of this book you will be provided a 6week proto- col as well as a recommended food list, but before you get to that part, there are some basic things to prepare for. Although you will be eliminating many foods and "foods" from your diet temporarily or full time, first focus on what you'll be adding in.

Veggies, especially high nutrient, organic greens need to be a huge focus at your main meals. I like to fill about half my plate with these types of veggies, not only to give me amazing fiber and energy, but also to fill my belly with bulk. You should never starve your body. It's important to remember this when making significant life changes.

Morning smoothies start your day off right. When you get into the habit of blending these up first thing each day, you'll be nurturing your body and your mind without even thinking about it. This has a substantial effect on how the rest of your day will go! I have provided a couple of my favorite smoothie recipes in this book but feel free to experiment. Remember you need a healthy base (nut milk, water, coconut water), healthy fat (coconut oil, chia seeds, avocado), optional fruit, optional protein and TONS of greens. Starting with these two tips will make this process smoother for you and start you off with an excellent amount of nutrition designed by nature.

Other key components of balancing your gut will be removing allergenic and toxic foods, adding healthy probiotic sources, discriminate use of supplements, healthy self-perception, stress control and adequate sleep. Instead of focusing on what you are removing, focus on what you are creating. You have chosen to create a healthy, vibrant body and mind. And because you have made that decision, all that's left is to nurture the body accordingly while it does its job.

Four

FOOD SENSITIVITIES AND ALLERGENS

There are a wide range of allergies and intolerances.
When it comes down to it, an individual could be sensitive to a number of things in their foods and environment, home, animals etc. This is why an "elimination and focus" regimen like the one outlined in chapter 13 is so critical. It allows you to pull common allergens and toxic substances from your consumption as well as your environment so that you may restore your gut and your well-being. Doing this while staying "in tune" to your body will allow you to strengthen your gut lining while making you aware of the things that it really doesn't like.

After balancing your gut, you may be able to tolerate some of the previously removed foods at different degrees, so keeping a journal throughout this process will make navigating those foods much easier. The most common allergenic whole foods are dairy, wheat/gluten and peanuts. Eggs are also common irritants but we have allowed farm fresh varieties during this period. If you think you have an issue with eggs, please choose not to consume them while you follow this plan.

Other irritants include soy, legumes and corn. Due to their high glycemic load (how fast a food turns to sugar) we have asked you to remove all grains. Quinoa is the one exception to the rule, due to its high fiber content, low allergy profile and lower glycemic load. It is technically a seed. We exclude legumes from the initial portion of this process because beans and legumes contain Phytic acid, which although fine in moderation, can bind to the nutrients in the food making them much less nutritionally beneficial. Another reason legumes are excluded is because they contain Galacto-oligosaccharides, which is a hard to digest carbohydrate for many people, especially those with digestive problems. I do encourage the trial of properly prepared beans and legumes during the reintroduction period. Testing how the body responds to different legumes may reveal a new tolerance to their occasional consumption.

Once the four weeks is through, you will start a reintroduction approach, where you will experiment with one whole food every four days and see how your body responds. This is when it will be especially helpful to journal throughout the day about your body and mood. Your body will react in different ways to different foods, so knowing what to look for will be essential.

Common signals that the body is having an allergic response include:

Digestive issues: Gas, bloating, irregular elimination patterns, heartburn and stomach upset. After feeling "clean and lean" during the elimination portion, it will become much more obvious to you when your digestive system is acting out like a toddler throwing a temper tantrum, ranging from mild bloating to full blown intestinal anarchy!

Skin changes: Acne, dryness, rashes and eczema are common to see. The skin is the body's largest organ and all organs are effected by a leaky gut. You just so happen to wear this particular organ across your face, so read it like a book! Often psoriasis and eczema are directly related to a gluten intolerance. I have known a few parents who have removed this one substance from their children's foods and watched their skin abrasions disappear.

Mood changes: This one is huge for me. After a month without any alcohol whatsoever, I chose to drink 1 beer. Just one. That was a bad choice not only due to the sugar and chemical content, but because of the high concentration of wheat. For two solid days, I felt incredibly agitated and restless and couldn't figure out why. That's where journaling comes in handy because that one beer was the only thing I had done differently in a month.

Energy: Feeling lethargic, exhausted or even manic are notable bodily communication. If you throw the wrong oil in your car, you can expect for it not to run right and probably sound kind of funny too. You are your best machine. If you aren't running right, then you possibly filled your tank with the wrong fuel.

Headaches and pains: We get too used to popping a pill at the first sign of a pounding head without considering the cause. My husband's headaches usually mean one of four things; he hasn't drunk enough water, his spine is out, he's lacking sleep or he ate something he shouldn't have. Achy and stiff joints can signal intolerance as well so if you go from feeling pretty agile to creeping out of bed like you need a walker, food could be the cause.

Allergy like/cold symptoms: Watery eyes, stuffy nose and a dry irritated throat are things to be aware of. Environmental toxins can produce reactivity like this too, so do note if you have come into contact with any harsh cleaning agents, fertilizers or body products.

Water retention, swelling, puffiness: Different things may cause you to retain water. If you notice a difference in the fit of your clothing overnight, or a noticeable puffiness under your eyes, in your face, hands or legs, consider what you have consumed. Fluctuations can occur due to things such as hormones and salt intake as well but after a while you will know your body enough to decipher the reason for these symptoms.

How are so many people allergic to "healthy" foods?

Humans weren't made to be so intolerant to whole foods. Allergies have become so predominant in our culture, largely due to two things, one being leaky gut. When the gut is overly permeable, food particles make their way into the blood stream, an area of the body they would not have otherwise seen. So even common foods like eggs or whole unprocessed wheat can now cause major inflammation by running awry outside the gut. The human body was originally designed to retain food particles within the digestive tract only. This allowed the absorption of nutrients and then elimination. With so many people suffering from leaky gut now days, negative reactions to everyday foods are a common result. Because of this however, once the gut is healed, some foods may become tolerable once again.

The second cause for food intolerance is GMOs. GMO's are the result of spliced DNA. A process where the genes of a plant or animal are combined with the genes of an unrelated species such as a bacteria, viruses, insects, animals or even human genes. This process results in what I have called "frankinfoods" or "foods" that never existed in nature. The goal of this splicing is to achieve effects that were difficult or unobtainable in the natural plant or animal such as withstanding the application of herbicides. Many GMO's even produce their own insecticide.

Genetically Modified Organisms are banned in the majority of developed nations. So why then does the US insist they are safe? Most likely due to the "trials" showing they are safe for human consumption. Ironically and not surprising, these trials are done mainly by the corporations creating the product in the first place. That's like asking my children to monitor and control their sugar intake in a free for all candy store!

Most livestock are fed GMO corn and soy products. Livestock that were originally meant to consume grass and bugs. In the documentary "King Corn", one farmer explains that on a diet of corn, a cow will not live past six months. Because cattle were not meant to consume corn and soy, it will take only six months for this diet to kill them. Since they are slaughtered before that, the industry pays no regard to this fact and Americans keep consuming sickly animal protein.

GMO's have only been around for a short while. They entered our food supply in 1994 in the form of the "flavor savor tomato". Since then, GMO's can now be found in most processed foods. The time span of which these foods have been in the American diet has not been long enough to truly know the consequences of consumption. The current pre-millennial generation has basically become the test subjects of chemical, scientifically produced "food". Even in this short duration, we still have enough information to connect food sensitivities to GMO's. Many people with an intolerance to say soy, may be able to tolerate an organic, non-GMO variety. With what we know about the body's immune system, we can be certain that feeding ourselves these unknown, unnatural substances is a surefire way to rev up an attack on our gut.

Although you may find yourself able to tolerate certain foods after the elimination period, you may choose to keep some out indefinitely. Knowledge is power and once you know the line that our modern food system has crossed, it may be hard to consciously impact your body so negatively.

Keeping your food organic and as close to home as possible is an excellent way to stand against GMO's and processed foods as well as supporting your local farmer and economy.

Five

THINK IT IN YOUR MIND, FEEL IT IN YOUR GUT

*H*ave you ever heard a song or driven by a certain place that brought back a strong memory? Whether it was good or bad, can you remember how you felt, literally? Where in your body do you feel your emotions? From time to time life gives us a little nudge into the past. When this happens we somewhat "re-live" that moment emotionally and physically; the reason why we hold onto that mix disc from our summer in San Diego, which when listened to brings back a nostalgia, or why we can't stand the smell of a fragrance worn by someone associated with a negative memory. The body feels our thoughts and sometimes stores emotions deep within our subconscious.

Researchers in Finland conducted a study of 700 participants and asked them to focus on 14 different emotions. The study required them to color in a chart of the body, showing where they felt activity and where they felt the absence of it. The results varied a bit from person to person but still showed similarities. I find this study compelling not because of the similarities but because of how easy it seemed to be for all those people to connect those emotions to their physical body. I recommend trying this yourself. Imagine a time when you felt extreme joy or sorrow, or fear. Note where in your body you feel energy from that feeling. Doing exercises like this will help you become aware of the physical responses to the things you feel, while strengthening your mind/body connection.

The mind/body connection is no joke. The only reason we feel pain is because the brain receives information from the inflicted area of the body via nerve fibers and thus interprets that as pain. On the reverse, when we see someone yawn, we often yawn ourselves, calling this a "contagious" reaction. This is why the term "mind-body connection" is used so frequently, especially in the holistic community. Understanding the connection between your mind and body is crucial to balancing your gut.

Ninety percent of the body's serotonin is produced in the gut. With mental illness climbing at rapid rates, this knowledge is very important. The subject of mental illness hits home for me as I myself had suffered with anxiety and depression for years. I have also watched many loved ones and friends be consumed with these horrible afflictions, only to blame themselves and shut themselves off from the world. Not only is the person with the illness suffering, more often than not so are the ones around them. A child with a depressed parent does not get the best of their loved one and can often pay long term for the experiences endured during their childhood.

Children with depressed parents often show signs of depression themselves but more often show defiant behavior such as acting out at school or home, appetite problems, anxiety, sleep issues and are more apt to have chronic depression in their teens and into adulthood. As sad as this is, most parents would never wish their ill health to affect their children. It is just an unfortunate side effect of a situation that already feels hopeless. This is why the gut-brain connection is so huge! It gives hope. Along with counseling and physical activity, healing the gut has the power to heal what pharmaceutical anti-depressants have only masked. The gut has intense power over the well-being of the mind, and the mind has power over the gut which is why Buddha belly focuses on a healthy mind-body approach to balancing both.

Of all the science that exists around the concept of mind-body, I feel it is important to speak freely and REAL regarding this topic. All the scientific explanation in the world won't make you more intuitive or self-aware. To really tap into your mind-body, you need to be able to quiet your mind and your surroundings enough to hear what your body is communicating to you.

Your body speaks to you constantly. Time to start listening

As we previously discussed, listening to the body's physical communication regarding the effects of foods and substances, as well as listening to the emotional ques it sends you, are equally important. Depending on the person, this awareness may come easily or be rather difficult.

Myself being an intuitive, deep thinking personality, I never understood how self-awareness could be so foreign to some. Then I attended my first real, professional counseling session. My counselor did an amazing job of dissecting my emotions and behaviors leading me to many new understandings of myself and my root feelings. This experience humbled me into the realization that although I am very deep and self-analyzing, there were parts of myself that I had not understood or even identified. Areas where I "shot in the dark", so to speak about my emotions and where they resonated from. I had tied certain feelings or behaviors to specific "reasons" and thus hadn't dug deeper. Through quality, professional therapy and my own openness, I now see life much differently.

It's hard to come to a realization such as I did, and not change. A little humility goes a long way. You may not feel that you have anywhere to budge, I feel that true personal evolution occurs once you're able to acknowledge that you will be forever evolving. Resisting humble self-awareness will only stunt the growth of your soul, thus holding you back from life.

Your inner voice

Your soul has a lot to tell you, and it uses your emotions to do so. Emotional reactivity is like a string tied to a phantom object. That object being a box that holds something essential to the soul's growth. For instance, the woman who holds a disdain for a woman who happens to be more educated then herself, regardless of how friendly that woman is, could benefit greatly from identifying the true reason behind that emotion. If she chose to acknowledge her negative thoughts toward the other woman, she might ask herself exactly what it is she is feeling? And why does she feel this way? The answer may be surprising to this woman. Maybe she feels insecure when around someone she perceived to be "smarter" then herself. Maybe this insecurity comes from a personal regret, or being berated in this area by someone she cared about like a parent or loved one.

Once we make these connections, we grow. We become aware of our weaknesses and our scars instead of hiding or ignoring them only to let them smolder and perpetuate our insecurity. This acknowledgment leads us to healing. Although healing our emotional wounds benefits those we come in contact with by eliminating the unconscious lashing out, even more, it benefits us. Negative feelings and thoughts come from a place of hurt. Your body wants to thrive in ALL areas including your soul. Negativity is a venom that first poisons our insides and then carries on to poison those within our reach. When you heal the holes in your heart, you will live happier and healthier.

True health is mental, emotional, spiritual and physical. Once you have tackled the food part, it is important to focus on your mind-body health by cleaning up your thoughts. Since emotions are relative, meaning they are what you make them, you can control a majority of the energy that is dispersed throughout your body, or at least the extent of its effect. Along your wellness journey you will be faced with many emotions; body image, self-confidence, faith, determination, fear, etc. Learning how to handle these moments will empower you through your personal transformation.

Your mind has the ability to affect the way you see life

Become VERY aware of your thoughts and feelings. What goes through your head when you think about your accomplishments, identity, body and challenges? What do you think/feel when you are around a variety of people similar or different then yourself? If journaling helps you with this process, then please write it down. Each day if you have to, reflect on the day and journal all your thoughts and emotions in any given situation.

"The truth will set you free"! Be honest with yourself. The only way to heal the root of your pains and emotions is by being candid about where they are buried and the signals they are sending out. I hate to break it to you, but we all have our own skeletons and our own kind of "crazy". I believe that the people who judge others the most, actually have the most digging to do within themselves. So, have no shame. You are becoming a better, healthier person as we speak and let me be the first to tell you from the bottom of my heart, I AM PROUD OF YOU!

I have two exercises or techniques that I routinely give people who are struggling with common worry, self-esteem issues or negative thoughts in general. The first is the 2 pound rule and the second is the "I AM" ritual.

The 2lb rule is when I coach someone to become aware of their thoughts and emotions in three categories: positive, negative and neutral. Positive thoughts consist of happy thoughts, optimistic feelings, or uplifting thoughts and feelings about others or yourself. Negative thoughts are those which put down or criticize others or oneself, view situations pessimistically (glass half empty) and anything that has a general negative tone. Neutral feelings and thoughts are observational such as "the sky is blue" or "that person is sad". Neutral thoughts have no intention, positive or negative, and don't invoke much of an emotional response.

Now I must state that I strongly dislike our society's constant obsession with weight. I find the focus on the scale to be misleading when practicing strength training activities (muscle weighs more than fat), taunting while trying to focus on patience through your transformation and berating to one's self-worth in general. However, because most people I work with are desiring improvement in this area, especially women, this technique works well.

Imagine that each thought you have, of yourself and others, will affect your weight on a scale. For every negative thought, you will weigh 2lbs more then you did before that thought and adversely, for every positive thought, you will lose 2lbs physical weight. For neutral thoughts, your weight stays the same. Take a moment to really receive this idea. Envision your body being an obvious indicator of your thoughts and judgements, especially towards yourself. Next, implement it into your daily life. Practice using this technique next time you look in the mirror or find yourself in a social situation. Not only will this provoke your self-awareness, it will also invoke an increase in positive thoughts and behaviors while helping bring more peace and less judgement into your daily living.

The "I AM" card is another affirmation and identification based strategy. Once you start focusing on your true emotional roots and their origins, you will be able to name many of your greatest fears and insecurities. The reason this is so crucial is because once you discover the negativity in your thought patterns, you can start to reverse it. The subconscious mind controls so much of our lives and truly believes everything it's told. If you tell yourself you are stupid or ugly, the subconscious holds onto that like a sponge, transforming how you see and feel about yourself into exactly what you have articulated. Letting fears constantly roam your mind will have a similar effect also, causing you to behave in a way that can end up manifesting those fears.

I like to use the example of the person with a strong attachment to a fancy car. How many times have you seen that individual nervous about door dings or damage, park at the far end of a parking area, only to have someone clip their bumper while every other vehicle was left unscathed? This goes hand in hand with the law of attraction. What you put out, you will receive. Projecting positive thoughts and handling fears in a healthy fashion will allow less of the things you fear into your life.

To start, fake it till you make it!

Speak what you desire the outcome to be and against your fears. Using the "I AM" card is an easy way to implement this strategy. Firstly, write down your top five biggest fears and insecurities on one side of a (two column) piece of paper. For example, "I am insecure about my body", "I am afraid of being alone", "I am not good enough at my job". Then in the other column, write down the opposite of the first column, for instance "I am insecure about my body" = "I am confident about my body and feel healthier everyday". Once you have filled out the reverse column, print only the positive affirmations on a small card. Keep this card easily accessible in a safe place like a wallet. Pull it out and recite these affirmations daily; multiple times a day if you need to. Whenever you feel overwhelmed by one of these burdening fears or unhealthy thoughts, just use the card. Your head will catch up to what it is you speak and in return will heal your heart.

Six

Stress is killing you

*"You should sit in meditation for 20
minutes each day, unless you are too
busy, then you should sit for an hour"*

- Old Zen proverb

The average person knows that stress isn't healthy. I find that most people I talk to agree that stress is just as much of a culprit behind disease as poor diet. However, knowing and doing are two separate things. It's always easier to put off until tomorrow what should be done today, until tomorrow never comes and the damage becomes extensive.

Stress comes in multiple forms but scientists have categorized it into three different types: acute, episodic and chronic. Acute stress is a short duration of stress and can be positive or negative. Being very excited about a presentation for work, or "jazzed" about a business idea or vacation is acute stress, as is being nervous about that same presentation or flight and just wanting it to be over with. This type of stress tends to only last momentarily. Acute stress can cause a range of symptoms from anxiety and irritability to stomach issues and more.

Episodic stress is similar to acute stress but in a frequent form. An individual who makes the same stressful commitments on a reoccurring basis might experience episodic stress. Unlike chronic stress, episodic stress ceases from time to time but remains a frequent occurrence. "Type A" personalities are a great example of this type of stress because a constant need for organization, control and sense of competition causes them to create their own reoccurring stress. Symptoms of this type of stress range from a constantly worried and highly agitated, manic state of being, to long bouts of depression.

Lastly, we have chronic stress. Chronic stress is by far the most damaging of them all and only consists of negative stress from unhealthy situations. Abusive relationships, unfulfilling careers and toxic home environment will create a state of chronic stress. Chronic stress happens when miserable life circumstances seem unrelenting and hopeless. The effects of chronic stress are almost endless. Some common signs are headaches, stomach aches, pounding heart, anxiety, depression . . . the list goes on. Although all forms of stress need to be monitored, chronic stress poses the most damage to our bodies, our well-being and especially our gut.

Life in general plays a part in all areas of the stress we experience. Some contributions are in our control while others have been bestowed upon us, with or without our consent. Take childhood for instance. When an infant enters this world, they are like a sponge and despite a parent's best efforts, that sponge will absorb everything it comes in contact with, forming who and what that infant grows into as an adult. Nobody's childhood was perfect but some have been dealt a shorter stick than others in this area. The effects of chronic, unrelenting stress, is deadly to the healthiest of adult bodies. Imagine what this type of stress can do to a vulnerable child.

In his book "*When the body says no*", Dr. Gabor Mate catalogs his time spent working with patients on end of life care. He draws specific ties between severe disease and stress, mainly in the form of chronic stress. He interviews many of his patients about their life experiences and their emotional coping styles. Many of his patients could be classified as chronic stress sufferers; people who were unable to draw healthy boundaries for themselves or who were subjected to traumatic childhoods consumed by fear and lacking a sense of control. A heavy number of the patients referenced in his book are those dying of cancer or other severe diseases such as ALS and many of them are astonishingly young. He does an excellent job of making you think. Hearing about a 22yr old woman with small children, dying of cancer, is enough to wrench your heart and stop anyone in their tracks. We can't change the past, but we deserve the opportunity to heal ourselves so that we can experience a healthier future.

Evaluating your stress

Who we are today is a culmination of a whole life's worth of experiences. Just as it is important to pay attention to our emotions and thoughts, we must also acknowledge our stress as well. Doing so will allow you to differentiate between unhealthy coping mechanisms (responses to stress) and truly unhealthy aspects of your life. Basically, is it your job that is stressing you out, or is it you who is creating the stress which will ultimately follow you wherever you go? When we pay attention to this part of living, we become much more present and able to navigate healthier habits for our daily lives. Not only does doing so cause you to feel more peaceful, it also brings a calm state to the body, aiding in a healthier functioning physical self.

If you need an example of this, just look at our presidents. The age progression throughout their time in office is a testimony to what I can only assume is stress related, accelerated aging. Most likely it's brought on by lack of sleep, poor quality of nourishment and excessive stress. It has been debated as to whether or not stress can cause the hair to turn grey, however I think that the examples speak for themselves.

A little science about stress

The science behind stress is compelling. When our body experiences the feeling of stress, it goes to work. The hypothalamus receives the body's threat signal and relays that to the nervous system which gets the heart pumping, lungs breathing and the stomach going. Stress literally affects your gut immediately, as well as long term. While in a state of stress, digestion is among many things hindered so that all the energy can go toward adrenaline or the "fight." A whole host of functions slow way down to allow the body to produce the immediate physical response necessary to escape perceived dangers. You can probably see why a frequent or constant state of stress can absolutely age and hinder the body. It's not being allowed to perform its functions fully for long periods of time and on top of that it is being overtaxed with adrenaline and cortisol.

Cortisol is a word that most people probably associate with belly fat. We hear it mentioned in commercials selling diet pills and articles about stress in our favorite magazines. It is a hormone produced by the body in response to stress. But did you know that cortisol has also been linked to memory malfunction, bone density problems, blood pressure, weight and more? It has shown a strong tie to depression and lower life expectancy. A recent study even showed a link between elevated cortisol and mental illness, especially in adolescence. Cortisol builds in the blood for the purpose of "fight or flight", but without the normal sequence that nature intended, such as running from an animal, cortisol just builds in the blood causing damage to the whole body. We are experiencing the destruction of our own bodies due to the very survival mechanism that was designed to save our lives. And for the most part, we only have ourselves to blame.

A lack of balance in the areas of work, play, health, personal time, creative time and relationships has become the "norm." Sunday's used to be a day of rest, and home cooked family dinners around the table were a staple of many households. Now, grabbing fast food to eat in the car while off to another scheduled commitment has taken the place of what used to be valuable quality time. Time to engage with your family over a nourishing meal provided not only connection, but consistency. This change has been the unfortunate outcome of traded time. Time is a highly valuable thing in this life, along with health and love, all of which don't come with a price tag. Well, that's not exactly true. We trade time for money every day; hours of our life in exchange for monetary wealth.

Living to work

As of March 2016, the average work week per person in the United States is 34.4 hours on the clock. Sounds normal, right? Except that average is just that, the average of all workers, both part-time workers such as students as well as overworked adults. In addition, the average commute time is 3.75 hours per week which puts us at an average of 38.15 hours per week working and commuting. Remember this is the average, which means most Americans are working much more then this! Then, add in all the fun home chores; laundry, cooking, cleaning, grocery shopping, all of which we will estimate at about 3 hours per day for 21 hours per week. Of the 168 hours in a week of our life, the average person donates 60 hours per week to just work and chores.

That leaves 108 hours left for sleep and life as we wish to make it. Since our bodies truly benefit from 8-10 hours of sleep a night (let's say 8), after work, chores and much needed rest, the average person is left with 52 hours per week or 7.43 hours per day. I like to call this time "Living time" because that's the hours you have for things outside of obligations and responsibilities. In the United States, of those hours an average of 4.56 hours are spent watching television or on media. This leaves us with 2.87 hours per day. No wonder we're stressed and depressed! The average person has under 3 house per day to get outside, perform physical activity, spend quality time with friends or loved ones or have any quiet time with their thoughts. Time, love and health. Remember? One might question if this is actually even living? For those who work more than the average, their "living time" is even less and they likely lack adequate sleep. You only have one life, and only one body to live it in.

What's it all worth anyway?

It is commonly stated that the American household cannot live on a single income. I'm not debating whether or not this is true for some, but I do feel that this perspective is highly subjective. Aside from those working minimum wage jobs, personal choices continue to dictate how much we "need" to work. Just like you added up your life time, (the time you spend working, cleaning etc.) you also need to add up how much of your work time is paying for needs verses just funding excess. Our basic needs include food, water, shelter, heat and clothing. Outside of these 5 basic necessities, there are then practical "needs" such as a vehicle to commute to a job that may be a significant distance away, or medical insurance. These things aren't necessities for survival but they are justifiable expenses. With that said, holding down a hefty car payment for a fancy new vehicle versus paying cash for a basic car that runs efficiently is where justifiable turns into excessive. Now don't get me wrong, there's nothing wrong with where one chooses to spend their money, and no one has the right to judge another. However, this is where we start adding up the cost of time.

Say you get paid for the 34.4 average hours worked per week and you make $12 per hour. This equates to $412.80 per week, minus 15% taxes, leaving you with $350.88 per week, or $10.20 per hour. Let's say that the payment for that new car is $350 per month, or $87.50 per week. Divide that by your hourly income and you will see that you work 8.6 hours per week just to pay for that car. The average person's work day is 6.88 hours per day, so technically you work about 1.25 of the 5 days just to pay for that car.

The purpose for laying out all the numbers this way is to help put into perspective what we trade our time for so that we can make conscious decisions regarding the disbursement of it. Remember back to the 7.43 hours a day that the average American has per day? Take away that car payment by purchasing a used vehicle and you now added 1.23 hours to your "Living time" equaling 8.66 hours per day. Start adding up credit card debt and the mortgage for a home that is more then what is needed for your family size and you'd have a heck of a lot more time! Maybe you could afford to work a job that is more enjoyable to you for less pay because you have mini-mized your expenses. We have choices. While one person may live minimally so that daycare for their children isn't needed, another may be comfortable working more in order to afford the vacation home that they enjoy with their family during their downtime. Conscious evaluation will allow you to make choices that you can be comfortable with and identify the areas of imbalance so that you can work toward putting them in alignment.

Finding a little joy in simplicity

I believe the soul resides in simplicity. That's why we feel at peace when in nature. When we live simply we are free to thrive in more *living* and less work. The more stuff you have, the more you need to work to maintain it, and the more time you must dedicate to cleaning and maintaining it. A good rule of thumb is "time or money?" Rarely are both an option. At the same time, each individual or family may have a differ-ent idea of what is enough and what is worth working for. For one person, a boat and all the expenses that come with it may be a ridiculous thing to trade time for especially depending on the average weather in their location. For another person, that same boat may be how they spend the majority of their free time and that provides a source of quality time with their family. They may sacrifice in many other less common areas in order to have this. The concept of "enough" is something that can only be navigated by you. This is your life, your time and your memories.

For me personally, I hate cleaning, especially dishes, but I need a clean house. My idea of "clean" has evolved since having children but I still have a hard time being peaceful in a cluttered or dirty home. My solution to these conflicting issues is to own a minimal amount of stuff. I have yet to achieve the level of minimalism that looks so amazing on all of my Pinterest boards, but it continues to evolve. I feel as though I am forever purging something. I have a fairly simple, versatile wardrobe, kitchen utensils and appliances that I absolutely use, and few clutter possessions. My preference is "I'd rather do, then have," meaning I'd prefer to get outside for a hike or even go out to dinner with a friend then buy stuff most of the time. Figuring out how to simplify in the areas that contribute to your stress will repay you handsomely in either more peace, time or money. Possibly all of the above.

"We could learn a lot from the distant world!"

Thankfully we are a species of comparison and when the world around us is out of sync, we seek examples of a better way, even if to just take notes. This can be hard to find in an industrialized, fast paced, "live to work" society. Fortunately for us, there are many groups of people around the world who have not "evolved" much from their ancestral roots. In John Robbins book "Healthy at 100" he documents his travels around the world to a few different groups of people. Generally, cultures living in isolation. Robbins documents the high amounts of centenarians amongst these people and details some of their daily life through his experiences while staying with them. He ties a lot of their health to diet but also touches on their lifestyle and community.

Many of these people work until they die, but not in the way we would assume. The goat herder for example, swiftly climbs the steep mountain well into his nineties, on a consistent basis, so that his goats may graze. The terrain is intense but his body is acclimated and his spirit is high. He enjoys the outdoors and doesn't possess the same job related stresses we associate with "work." He's diligent but not rushed. And in a world like this there is no such thing as "higher productivity." Most typical jobs are designed for productivity. The more you do in less time means more money, and when one goal is met, another is quickly set. Constantly focusing on achieving MORE is draining on the body and makes simple work related tasks much more stressful.

In small cultures, such as the ones referenced, the people often "work" for their food and well-being, not monetary compensation, and are often accompanied by friends, family or community all doing the same thing. Imagine if your job consisted of tending your garden and other necessary home needs while your spouse and children pitched in, and then you break to share meals together. Even though these are long days, the ambiance of these environments is much more peaceful and life giving then an American nine to five. Happiness was noted as being a contributing factor to the longevity of life in these regions as well as a highly alkaline diet and community.

In a world, full of technology, towers and heavy machinery, our bodies still crave simplicity to some degree. This is why when we envision a sandy beach or small cabin in the woods we feel a sense of calm. Noise and the constant bombarding of ads and media, while navigating five o'clock traffic, is enough to send your nervous system into overdrive and your cortisol levels through the roof.

Taking more "down time" where possible can help undo some of the damage modern living has inflicted. I often sit with no TV on and read a book while sipping tea, or do yoga in my designated chill space while listening to my favorite music. In these moments I feel peaceful and content and nothing feels healthier then peace. When in a peaceful or neutral state the body and mind have a chance to rest and rejuvenate. Making time for these life-giving moments will not only benefit your gut, but your entire health.

And then we meditate

Meditation is an incredible way to nurture your body and alleviate stress. Meditation is defined as "contemplation, thought, reflection or prayer." Taking quiet time to meditate has considerable effects on your health. In a Harvard study, meditation was shown to actually alter the brain by preserving it from aging, improving focus, reducing overall stress, encouraging creative thought, and rivaling pharmaceutical effects on anxiety and depression. It is astounding to see the quantity of studies done on such a conceptual practice. I have found science to loosely acknowledge things that don't swim in front of a microscope. These studies however do measure brain activity and behavior changes which are visible proof.

Meditation is a practice that has been around for centuries. Traditional meditation is usually associated with the Buddhist monks who were the first well documented practitioners of meditation. But some researchers speculate that it goes back to hunter gatherers who may have discovered this altered state while staring into the fire. It would be silly to mark a spiritual practice like this with a date of creation because it is a personal practice and experience that may look different for everyone. Although meditation is a strong part of the Buddhist faith, the very definition of meditation includes focused thinking and prayer in general. No matter what your personal belief system, you can find a place for meditation because it is a focused, quieting of the mind, or conscious control over thought. Take time to still the mind or direct your thoughts in a healing way, such as gratitude, affirmations or a good heart to heart with God. It is a nurturing moment. If you could hook up to a machine while doing this that would measure your heart rate, blood pressure and brain activity, you would see firsthand that the body needs this time and rejuvenates when given the opportunity.

If you are new to the concept of meditation, don't be intimidated. There is no "right" way, and the more you practice, the more natural it will become and actually addictive it can become. The addiction factor comes from experiencing how good it feels to be peaceful and alive. You will eventually learn to use this as a tool to combat a hard day or rough patch in life or even to just indulge yourself because it just so happens to be the healthiest way to do so.

Meditation isn't a place, it's a mental and spiritual experience and therefore can be done anywhere. However, I recommend making a cozy place in a corner of your home, or wherever you have space. A yoga mat or even a pillow is nice to sit on. You can use essential oils to help you relax, such as lavender, or play peaceful music or nature sounds as well. Try and make your meditation space simple and clean so that there are less distractions. Even if you have to face a corner and forget about the mess behind you, that will at least allow you to focus on the moment without the dishes intervening in your Zen.

Next, sit comfortably, relaxed and with straight posture. Practice breathing deeply and slowly while quieting mental chatter. Focusing on your breath will help distract you from a busy mind. Once you have calmed your mind, the rest is up to you. Maybe this is a chance to pray. Maybe you use this time to envision a sandy beach and ocean waves in order to entice the body into a peaceful state. Positive affirmations are a great addition as well. Start with five minute sessions and work your way up to what you feel is needed on each individual day.

If you are anything like me (a little "type a") you may find it difficult to make time for meditation, which probably means you are especially in need of it. During my coursework, one of my assignments was a month long self-nurturing practice of specialized eating and daily meditation. I had a far easier time with the restricted diet then I did with the daily meditation. As much as I wanted to, making time for me was incredibly difficult. I often forgot, or was so caught up taking care of the family that it didn't happen. All the while my body craved more self-nurturing.

Months later I made a decision. I had let my life get way too off balance. My husband's work priorities and the needs of my three kids had taken a majority of my time and although blessed, I was getting irritable and in need of a little peace. That's when I decided to start my month of meditation. I made a time each day during which the baby would sleep, where I would meditate. What this month taught me was priceless. I couldn't alter the circumstances or my priorities at the time; in fact, five minutes each day was sometimes all that I got to myself. But I could make that time count. I referenced this experience in the Testimonials chapter because for me, the experience effected my state of well-being just as much as my eating habits had. Loving yourself enough to nurture your body from the inside out will alleviate the burden that stress has inflicted and allow positive growth to occur naturally.

Seven

LOVING YOURSELF AND
NURTURING YOUR BODY

You can't nurture something you despise

Loving you and appreciating your body is so important on a true health journey, especially while awaiting results. I like people to think of their physical body like they do their children. Could you imagine telling your child that their little baby rolls are "gross", or looking at your teen dressed up pretty for prom and saying "If only you could lose another ten pounds, maybe you wouldn't see those love handles". Or how about men: would you say to your growing son "you won't be good enough until you look like that guy". Absolutely not! The negative repercussions to their self-esteem and confidence would be insurmountable! Yet, we talk to ourselves like this every day. Every time we stand in the mirror and criticize what we see or put ourselves down in public or alone, we are berating our inner self. This behavior teaches your sub-conscious to believe the negativity and ultimately manifest it, resulting in depression, stress low self-esteem and eventually costing you your physical health.

No amount of makeup, perfect clothing, muscles or weight loss will ever give you true confidence or self-esteem. This can only come from a deep appreciation and understanding of yourself and a desire to nurture your body out of love. Loving yourself and your body doesn't mean that you have to be happy with everything about it. It means you love yourself at the soul level and understand that the physical part is just a result of the level of nurturing you've done. Your physical body should be used as tool for measuring how well you have loved yourself thus far. View extra weight as a symptom because it is. Your weight has nothing to do with who you are; nothing about your body does.

It is important to distance your emotions with regard to awareness of your physical attributes. They are all markers of your life, both good and bad. Extra body weight often indicates challenges with diet and lifestyle, yes, but deeper issues such as self-medicating emotional wounds and stress are also to blame. In order to heal this area, we need to heal the root cause that is contributing to the symptom of excess weight, and you can't get to the root if you are busy feeling self-conscious about the symptom. At the same time, the nose that you dislike was passed on by many others before you. Relatives who had an impact, even if indirectly, on your journey. Embrace your unique traits by affirming their beauty for what they stand for. Your traits tell your story. Accept the weight on your body as part of your life up to this point and have peace with it knowing that at this moment you are evolving and changing for the better.

Some physical changes such as those left from childbirth can be significant, but they are a reminder that you carried life within your body. I find this area to be the biggest struggle for most women I talk to. Pregnancy sometimes leaves changes in the skin as well as weight that, despite one's best efforts, may never be what it was pre-baby. As frustrating as this may feel, trust that by nurturing your body with life giving foods, healthy activity and positive environments and thoughts, your body will align itself right where it needs to be. A healthy weight for you, with strength, energy and happiness. Doesn't that sound amazing? Feeling content in your skin is only part of it. Once you let go of a self-perceived "ideal" image, you can relax and actually enjoy your healthy body, because a healthy mind will accompany it. And generally, you will look great to the world around you as well.

If only we could all view health in the same light. One of the most disheartening things about being a health coach in this current world is the subliminal messages that perpetuate self-hate. In a world more concerned about perfect abs then cancer prevention or self-esteem, it makes pioneering true health that much more difficult. I define *True Health* as a balanced state of well-being, mentally and emotionally as well as physically. Mentally you should feel neutral and peaceful a majority of the time, with an ability to focus when necessary, and most of your thoughts should be of a positive nature. Emotionally, you should feel even keeled and be capable of expressing yourself healthily, while also knowing when to seek professional help in areas that feel consistently hard to tackle.

Even a healthy person won't handle life's situations like this all the time, but a balanced person will possess these character traits more often than not, as well as a desire for further self-growth. Perfection will never be achieved in anything so don't let that interfere with your positive stride. Some days I look at my life and how I think and act and I see how truly far I have come. Other days (usually a rough day when I wasn't my best) I feel as though I'm back where I started. This isn't true though. In those moments when you feel as though you have back pedaled, it is more often a sign that you are more aware of your state of being now and you desire to be better then you have been before. That is progression.

Lastly, the aspect of physical health. When your physical body is healthy you should experience level energy throughout your day, quality sleep, rare sickness, good skin, healthy digestion and elimination, and of course a healthy weight that is optimal for your body. Now this is where it gets tricky. Many people, especially women, chase the weight part of health when in reality, weight is just one of many symptoms of health. By solely focusing on this one aspect, you are neglecting all the other areas of health. Far too often a quest for a physical weight or body image leads people to partake in things that are actually quite harmful to their true health and their gut. Restricting calories, over exercising, using diet supplements and even surgery are often used to create an ideal physique. These practices rob you of true health and usually lead to compulsive behaviors, making a state of peace unobtainable.

Nobody is the same, however, everybody needs nurturing. You need to eat, move and rest. Failing to treat your body right will result in a decreased state of overall health and usually fail to deliver the superficial results desired in the first place. Over exercising can be a form of self-abuse and is considered a disorder under certain circumstances. There was a point in my life where I can remember spending two hours on a piece of exercise equipment in an attempt to burn every calorie I'd eaten that day. Not only was that irrational and unhealthy but it also slowed my metabolism by decreasing my muscle mass, causing my body to hold onto fat much easier thereafter.

Throw away your scale

Focusing on weight as a marker of health is as silly as paying thousands of dollars for a car with a pretty paint job without checking the engine. It's impractical, and yet we live in a society that encourages this misguided preoccupation. Why? Because business makes a lot of money off our insecurities and naivety in regards to actual health! The amount of money spent annually on diet programs and products is huge, and yet the health of the nation is on a consistent decline. I believe this is mainly due to two reasons. One is that people want a quick fix, which causes them to seek diet products with simple promises, while degrading their long-term health in the process. Secondly, the average person is uneducated about what true health actually looks and feels like, so they get caught up in what media and manufacturers paint it to be.

Don't be offended by this. Large food operations and product manufacturers go to extensive lengths to mislead the public's understanding of what's safe and healthy. Navigating through the garbage could be a fulltime job. I personally feel that no one should ever take a diet or appetite pill. Aside from being potentially very dangerous, most are ineffective. No pill or product will teach you how to eat and live in a nurturing way, nor will they give you the tools to a lifetime of true health. True health is only possible when you make the choice to love and focus on all aspects of yourself, not just your weight.

What does your best body look like?

At age 31, it finally clicked for me. It literally took that many years for me to figure out that instead of telling my body what it should look like and trying to manipulate it to fit that ideal, I needed to sit back and focus on nurturing my body in all areas and let it tell me what ideal looked like for me. Odd concept, isn't it? The need for control can be so counterintuitive for our well-being. Sometimes giving up control allows for acceptance to transcend into peace. This becomes possible when we direct our actions toward nurturing health. By providing your body, without restriction, everything it needs to thrive, it easily will. Now it is up to you to appreciate the outcome. Don't get me wrong, if you want to do some focused strength training so that your biceps look nice or your booty fills out your jeans better, be my guest. But no physical goal should come at a price. Ignoring the body's need of rest or nourishment in the name of a leaner you, is not true health. Comparing yourself to others or sacrificing balance will only send you backwards from how far you have come.

Everyone has a different body type and if each person focused first on balancing their gut health as well and their true health, the outcome would still look different for everyone. Some people will gain muscle or lose fat easily while others may struggle a little more. Just because the best you may not look like what you strove for up until now, it is a beautiful body that now comes with a healthy state of being. With that said, you might be surprised at just what the final product of you actually looks and feels like. The best you might out do your previous expectations. Enjoy the visible improvements while you continue to progress in other areas.

You should notice clearer skin, and healthier hair and nails. One of the most encouraging improvements in the beginning of balancing your gut is the lack of bloat, caused by improved digestion. This may come at different times for different people. Some individuals will experience bloating until their bodies become accustomed to the increase in beneficial bacteria from the probiotics, as well as increase in fiber consumption. During the initial phase, you will likely experience some form of "detox" symptoms. When your body detoxes from things such as sugar, it can be a rough experience. Symptoms like lethargy, runny nose, odd cravings and irritability are common but will clear up once your body kicks out the junk. These discomforts are no reason to re-feed yourself these substances. The withdrawal symptoms are your body's way of cleansing itself from foreign chemicals and toxins. Soon enough you should feel "cleaner" and more energetic. At that point the road gets smoother because it is much harder to put junk into your body once you experience how amazing healthy feels.

Pack the magazines away with the scale

Focusing on superficial images can be discouraging. I personally find "fitspiration" (sites and pictures of men and women in competition shape) to actually do quite the opposite of motivation. I feel that these sites and blogs cause people to judge themselves even harder and distract them from focusing on their true health. I don't judge what someone enjoys focusing on or showing off but I understand the immense role of the subconscious and its effects on behavior and self-esteem. More often than not, images such as these evoke inadequacy rather than motivation, causing a myriad of negative self-talk which, as I've mentioned, will hold you back on this journey. I advise you to put away any kind of advertisements, media (including social media) and anything that tempts you to be critical of yourself. Criticism won't get you anywhere but depressed. The future best version of yourself needs to be uplifted and encouraged to blossom. A flower can't bloom in the dark, so in order to keep your mind right, avoid or limit anything superficial that doesn't give life to your true health. Rather than focusing on images of six pack abs and perfect thighs, instead set physical goals in the form of achievements, such as perfecting your yoga practice or improving your lifting technique. By directing your attention towards new exciting goals and activities, you'll strive for improvements in a positive light and your body's strength and physical form will follow suit.

Positive focus fitness and health is what I call this type of non-dieting, and it is honestly the easiest way to lose weight and improve body image. I consider the typical kind of "dieting" ("If I eat less and squat more, maybe I will like my body") negative focus dieting and fitness. It is easy to tell the difference between the two because one makes you feel great no matter where you currently stand and the other bullies you into exercise and eating as a form of self-abuse. This type of negativity tells you that you aren't good enough and only when you achieve (insert self-criticism here) will you be able to be happy. No wonder making positive strides with our health and weight can seem like an impossible dream! Apologize to yourself for all the times you've let this negative focus dieting treat your body and your mind like garbage and embrace a new way towards health through self-nurturing and positivity.

I believe most people, especially women, practice negative focus dieting and health. The interesting part about this is that it effects people of all shapes, sizes and ages. Regardless of the current state of a person's form, diet, or body fat percentage, their health could be severely lacking in this area. When I get a group of participants together for gut health groups, I love seeing a variety of people. Unlike most weight loss programs, I have men and women at all stages of life and with a diversity of bodies. After the program gets going, I love to see people relax with each other, realizing they are all there for the same reason no matter how different they may feel from one another. Each person is there to achieve their own true health. Each individual has recognized that something about their way of living is robbing them of experiencing true well-being. The person who you feel so inferior to may be struggling with severe insecurity and self-destructive behaviors, or miserable digestive distress. Now I am not a phycologist and I openly discuss the benefits of a good counselor when dealing with deep rooted issues, but I do play a big role in helping people self-analyze. Doing so is a major component in gut and life balancing.

Wear it like you love it, and don't forget to smile.

There is nothing more attractive then real confidence. The kind you see in people who just look comfortable wherever they go and however they look that day; the person who easily says hello with a smile and isn't intimidated by the environment around them. We are easily drawn to this kind of person for their energy, and that energy is attractive because it's a quality most people wish to have. There is however a fine line between confidant and conceited. Someone who is conceited may appear to be confidant but in reality, this is a show to cover up unresolved self-esteem issues. Someone who acts this way will usually spend a lot of time talking highly of themselves in an unconscious attempt to get you to see them in a certain light. If this person is you, then make sure to be aware of your self-talk so that you can encourage it in a healthy direction. Let people see you for who you are, not who you tell them you are, and have peace about the outcome. If your heart is in the right place, it will be obvious.

A smile goes a long way! When you think happy thoughts, that energy becomes apparent in your body language and your facial expressions. Have you ever had a better than average day and found yourself walking through a large group of people, only to receive unusual amounts of smiles, greetings and even compliments from total strangers? This happens because people are effected by the energy you give off. When you are happy and friendly, you are radiant and you attract that energy in return. This type of attractiveness is an excellent area to focus on while you are on your true health journey because it deflects your attention from your superficial traits and causes you to focus on who you really are and how you think.

Buddha Belly doesn't just focus on food and exercise. Gut balancing is just as effected by emotional stresses and negativity. Improving your microbiome will not be achieved if you focus only on what you put in your mouth and ignore what you allow in your head. You must transform from the inside out. Nurturing yourself with love needs to come before the physical changes will take place. Life is really short; too short to self-obsess or focus on things that bring you down. Once you understand this concept, the diet and lifestyle modifications will be easy. Remember to talk yourself up each day. Tell yourself in the mirror that you appreciate your body and what it's done for you and that from here on out you will nurture it so that you can enjoy a great quality of life together long into old age.

Eight

MOVE, HYDRATE, REST, REPEAT

A body in motion stays in motion. We are a species that was designed to move. Although the average person knows this, how to go about physical activity can feel daunting. One side of the spectrum touts excessive weight training as the "perfect" mode of health while the other side pushes you to be the next marathon runner. Physical activity is an enjoyable addition when following Buddha Belly's balancing plan. So, which form of exercise is the way to go?

Honestly this depends on a few things: where you currently are with fitness, your body type and most importantly, what you like! No matter how effective a certain form of exercise may be, if you don't enjoy it then you won't fully benefit from it. If you are counting down the minutes until it's over, then you won't be truly engaged in your activity causing you not to reap the full rewards. Evaluate where you are at this moment and take into consideration how your body is responding to your new eating habits. Don't be afraid to back off or change direction and follow another mode. Exercise should give you energy, not deplete it. If nothing else, just keep moving. Go for daily walks and stand as much as possible, like when doing computer work. The body is adaptable and the less time you spend sitting, the more fit you'll be.

How we were designed to move

From the beginning of time, humans were meant to move. With the goal of survival, physical activity usually consisted of a lot of walking, occasional sprinting, climbing, stretching and lifting. Because so much time was spent out in nature's elements hunting and gathering, this form of cross-training was just a natural part of everyday life. The benefit to this however was that it kept the body agile and fit in a way that few gym goers experience today. The heart and lungs were strong, as was the musculoskeletal frame, and bone density wasn't at all a problem. As with diet, I feel that we perform physical activity too often with the intention of altering our physical body instead of just using it to experience life or increased health. There are those who seek out forms of sports or certain hobbies like rock climbing, strictly for the enjoyment of the activity. These individuals benefit from the lack of stress involved with performing a task out of enjoyment, while also experiencing the physical benefits as well.

At one point during my coaching, I did a month of activity which ranged from heavy weights to hill training and basic walking with a stroller. I conducted this experiment over our social media site and titled it "Active April, throw away your scale." The purpose of this month was to take the focus completely off the dreaded weight tracking and try multiple different forms of activities. I joined a local women's strength training group, practiced high intensity interval training (HIIT) workouts on the hill by my house, isometric based DVD's, and even Arial yoga. I liked all of these workouts and was able to note which forms my body responded to best and which ones I enjoyed the most. One of the most enlightening discoveries for me personally was seeing that my body liked many different forms of exercise and possessed almost a need for certain workouts at certain times or on certain days. For instance, at the beginning of the week when I was the most rested, my strength training routine and my HIIT workouts were the most desired and successful. Mid-week was an excellent time for Yoga and stretching, and daily walking kept me loose. Listening to my body enabled me to give it what it needed and allowed me to appreciate all that it could do.

Although it may be awkward at first, seeing your body move in ways that it hasn't before gives you a new respect for it. Yoga is an excellent example of this. As you improve your practice, your flexibility and form improve. Yoga not only helps you feel peaceful, but it helps you feel sexy, much like dancing. Yoga is an almost artistic expression and can be done by just about anyone regardless of physical ailments or issues. During the beginning of the Buddha Belly program you may want to stick to subtle exercises such as yoga, especially if you are new to physical fitness or dealing with adrenal fatigue. This practice is easily tailored to each person no matter where they are while also providing a relaxing experience.

HIIT is a form of burst exercise. Sprinting, or heavy lifting (maxing out) for a short, hard period of time, is an example of HIIT exercise. This type of training is very effective for burning fat and is an efficient way to lean out the body with a short duration of intense activity. Football players practice a lot of HIIT based workouts. They sprint and tackle with full exertion followed by a period of rest before doing this again. Many experts state that this type of fitness is optimal for burning fat and will create the most desirable body.

Strength training is another form of fitness as well as an excellent way to build your musculoskeletal body. As long as proper form is used, isolated movements can be used to build specific muscle groups. This type of exercise is beneficial for the body's metabolic rate (rate at which it burns energy or calories). The more muscle mass you possess, the more calories you will burn on a constant basis. Strength training can mold the structure of your body and help even extra weight sit more flattering.

Like they say, "abs are made in the kitchen"

This is true. The majority of physical improvements will become visible with a nurturing form of eating. While fitness has a concrete space in our lives, it is much less effective when the body isn't being fueled and cared for properly. The functions responsible for how your body burns fat and builds muscle are very much effected by the degree of toxins bogging down your liver. Buddha Belly understands the connection between both of these elements which is why we emphasize the nurturing nutrition portion so strongly.

A great way to look at your body in regard to fitness is like a nice suit or dress. It is something you wear that dresses up what you already have on the inside. Despite your body fat percentage, your musculoskeletal frame is your Armani or little black dress. It is a suit designed solely for you and your frame. Performing exercise should firstly be enjoyable, and secondly it should be a way to tailor that unique outfit to your body. I find that it helps to focus on the body's structure, especially when new to fitness or starting a journey into health. It is far more common to focus on the outer layer of weight or undesirable traits then it is to focus on structure. Again, like with diet, we want to motivate our best self from the inside out, not bully it into existence. Because your body's structure is its support and truest form, focusing on building, stretching and appreciating it will distract you from negative criticism and allow you to see progress more clearly.

Progress comes in so many forms such as flexibility, speed, heart rate, stamina, strength, agility and balance. Focus on the positive improvements in these areas while listening to your body's communication. For some people, certain forms of activity such as intense lifting or excessive cardio may not be right for their body at a certain point in time. Only perform activities that suit your current state of fitness and progress slowly. Find motivation in everything from improved muscle definition to an increase in stamina. Get creative with your fitness and have solace in the fact that you are already nourishing your body in a new way which is more than half the battle.

You are what you drink

Anyone with a remotely green thumb knows that if you don't water a plant, it will not survive. But before its demise, it will wilt, slump over then the leaves and petals will fall off and eventually it will die. Our bodies are approximately 60 percent water. In a day in age where cola and energy drinks are regularly consumed and juice and chocolate milk are considered the "healthy" option, we are very dehydrated. When the body is lacking sufficient $H2O$, it can't function as intended. Water is essential for proper digestion, detoxification and proper vitamin and mineral absorption. When your hydration needs aren't met, symptoms such as fatigue, mood swings and headache are common and in severe cases, kidney malfunction and even death can occur. In an already under nourished population, do we really need to exacerbate this by ignoring our water needs? Seems ridiculous to me.

In recent studies, it was concluded that approximately 75 percent of Americans are chronically dehydrated and this is largely due to an over consumption of soda and similar beverages, as well as lack of whole, fibrous, water containing foods. Chronic vitamin and mineral deficiencies can come from many things, but chronic dehydration is a significant factor. By staying hydrated you can eliminate this common cause. It is recommended that the average person consume half of a gallon of water a day. An easy way to achieve this is to limit or omit any non-water based drinks. Infusing your water with berries and fruit or cucumber is a great way to dress it up. Herbal teas are caffeine free and as long as they aren't combined with artificial sweeteners, they are a healthy option as well.

Don't forget your beauty rest

The role that sleep plays in your life cannot be underestimated. Sleep has the ability to make or break you. Believe it or not, the average person needs eight to ten hours of sleep a night to reap the full benefits of bodily rejuvenation. The average adult currently gets around six and a half hours of sleep per night. Children need approximately nine to thirteen hours per night to support healthy growth and brain function. This may sound excessive but adequate rest is something you need to make time for.

A lot happens during the resting hours. The kidneys and liver work hard to detox that day's exposures and the digestive system focuses on processing nutrients. The body works on muscle and tissue repair, memory consolidation and the functions of hormones that have a multitude of effects on the body. According to the national sleep foundation, there are four stages of sleep. Stage one is light sleep or "half sleep." Stage two is the onset of sleep where your body temperature drops and your breathing and heart rate become regular. Stage three and four are the stages of deep sleep where the blood pressure drops, breathing slows, muscles relax, hormones are released and energy is restored. It is during this phase of sleep that your health is most affected. Interfering with the release of essential hormones has an effect on appetite control, hunger signals and growth. This can have very negative consequences on a child's development as well as an adult wishing to lose weight and build muscle.

Think of full, complete sleep like a dishwasher or washing machine. If you don't let it finish the cycle, you will likely get dirty dishes or clothes that are too wet to put in the dryer. By repetitively stopping your cycle short you are inhibiting your body from completing its healthy functions and working against your health goals. The important bacteria in your gut are even affected by your sleep. With gut health being the goal, it is important to prioritize sleep as part of your gut balancing journey. Scientists are finding that as much as the microbiome effects sleep function, improper sleep also effects the quality and diversity of gut microbes. Gut microbes are like skin cells, constantly dying while the body works to make new ones. Much of this process takes place during sleep, so when adequate sleep is not achieved it can affect the body's ability to replace the lost microbes.

Sleep is the new Botox!
Just as microbes are replaced during sleep, so are cells. With your skin being the largest organ of the human body, a lot of energy is needed to replace skin cells and repair damage. A lack of rest can age a person very quickly. Studies show

accelerated aging of the brain in individuals with poor sleep habits, as well as an increase in Alzheimer's disease. When a person is tired, the body releases more cortisol. The presence of cortisol deteriorates the collagen in the skin, making more lines and wrinkles. We count on the human growth hormones released during rest for strong bones, skin and muscle mass. Because multiple functions are performed during different stages of sleep, a full cycle of sleep is as crucial to your health as water, diet and exercise.

REM sleep stands for Rapid Eye Movement. REM sleep should occur for 25% of the evening starting about 90 minutes into sleep and occurring every 90 minutes lasting for longer durations as the night goes on. During REM sleep is generally when dreams occur. The brain is active but the body is limp and possibly "twitchy." Scientists still do not fully understand REM sleep. In one study, when rats were robbed of REM sleep for four weeks they died. According to an article in Scientific American, this could be because REM sleep is needed for regulating body temperature and neurotransmitter levels. They go on to state that "fetuses and babies spend 75 percent of their sleeping time in REM." Many psychologists believe that this stage of sleep has a purpose and that it consists of meaningful dreams.

Regardless of the unknown reasons for different stages of sleep, we have enough information to understand the importance of adequate, quality rest. To ignore this area of your health is selling yourself short. As the mother of a 9mo old, breast fed baby, I understand that there are forces beyond our control. That is why it is so crucial to make time to rest whenever possible. A mid-day cat nap can do wonders for your energy while helping make up for a night of poor sleep. Setting a "get ready for bed" time is a great way to wind the body down and ensure an earlier shut eye.

One big disruptor of sleep is technology. Television, computers, phones and artificial lights keep the body awake. Humans were never designed to live around artificial light. Prehistoric man made fire when light was needed and usually slept and woke according to the rise and fall of the sun. Strangely, light from fire does not have the same effect on the brain as artificial illumination. Blue lights and artificial illumination effect our biorhythms, the rhythms that are responsible for our sleep patterns. Too much "light" in the night hours, when the body is trying to wind down, confuses it into thinking that daylight is still present and therefore puts off its normal rest functions; functions which calm the body and mind, preparing it for restful sleep.

Blue light, or light that is omitted from technological devices, really affects the sleep rhythms and the body's production of melatonin, a hormone responsible for keeping you asleep. In order to set yourself up for sleep success, make a habit of being in bed by 10 pm each night. Most sleep rejuvenation is done between 1am and 3am. If you are waking during these hours, not only are you not getting restful sleep, but it is possibly a sign of a bogged down liver. During these hours is when a large amount of detoxification takes place and if the liver isn't functioning properly this could be apparent in sleep cycle disruption. Getting to sleep later than 11 pm, doesn't allow the body to get into the deep sleep necessary for the rejuvenation period by 1am.

Try some of these tips. At least one to two hours before bed, turn off all electronic devices and dim the lights. Try stretching or taking a hot Epsom salt bath to help you relax. Refrain from eating at least three hours before sleep and avoid alcohol. Alcohol is taxing on the liver and actually inhibits restful sleep. Sugar and other stimulants should also be avoided in the evening, and stay away from caffeine after 10 am. For those who suffer with insomnia and chronic fatigue, these avoidances may feel impossible. Relying on a cocktail at night to pass out and stiff coffee throughout the day to keep going is a vicious cycle that only perpetuates a vicious cycle. Sleep issues are a huge sign of leaky gut and although these sleep practices may feel difficult at first, they will pay off in the long run. A body and mind that are well rested will reward you with improved mood, hormonal function, and a quality immune system.

Make your bed a spa experience

Instead of looking at sleep as a stressful thing you don't have enough time for, or flopping into bed out of exhaustion at the end of the day, make your sleeping environment a peaceful experience. Think of how wonderful it feels to get a good massage. The room is usually dimly lit with low peaceful music or nature sounds and smells of essential oils. Design your bedroom in a way that promotes tranquility. Rub your feet with lavender oil and play some ocean sounds. Make sure your bed is cozy and your room is free of clutter. Spend time in your room or bed without technology before actually going to sleep. This is a good place to stretch, meditate, pray and practice calming your mind. The more you can wind down before actual sleep occurs, the less active your thoughts will become and the better quality your actual sleep experience will be.

Nine

KEEPING IT REAL:
HOME AND BODY PRODUCTS

*H*undreds of thousands of chemicals have been produced in the last two hundred years, making the full regulation of them almost impossible. The long-term effects of being exposed to all of these toxic substances is still so unknown. Just because the exact effects of any one chemical isn't certain, it is certain that many of these chemicals are responsible for the influx of cancer and other related illness. In one study, scientists found many toxic chemicals present in the DNA of children that were banned decades before the child's conception. This suggests that long after we "clean up the problem" these toxic substances are still saturated in our environment, only left to harm future generations.

Non-organic methods of growing food, has poisoned our food and our environment. If you have ever watched a small prop plane spray pesticides over a field of corn, you can imagine the quantity of toxic chemicals present in our air, doused on our food, and left to seep into our ground water. Buying organic whenever possible, especially when purchasing fruits and veggies, will help lessen your exposure. Buying directly from a local organic farmer is even better. Local, organic produce is the next best thing to growing your own food. It enables you to consume food shortly after it is harvested and most operations will be happy to give you a tour of their farm and let you see for yourself how the food is grown and treated.

What good is a clean toilet if it gives you a weak gut?

Household cleaners, chemicals and beauty products are crammed into the average person's cupboard. There are specific products for everything. One product is for the toilet, the other is for the sink and then there is the floor cleaner which might be next to the glass spray; each individual concoction promising to help make your life easier and your home spotless. What these products fail to mention is that along with a squeaky-clean countertop, you will also be exposed to a long list of chemicals and their side effects.

The most toxic chemicals found in the average home consist of anti-corroding products: oven cleaners and toilet cleaners. Although these are the highest toxicity, it's the everyday "low toxicity" products that add up over time. Because these low-tox products are used so frequently, the low levels of chemicals build up in the body. Then there's the fact that multiple different products contain the same chemicals, so in one day you are easily exposed to these toxic substances again and again.

Some concerning ingredients found in everyday products (mainly body products) are parabens, which are a form of preservative used to prevent bacterial growth. Parabens mimic estrogen and have been found in breast cancer tumors. They are currently used in many different products but are very common in beauty products and shampoos. Phytates are used to create flexibility in plastic substances and are linked to endocrine disruption and cancer. Triclosan is another ingredient used as an anti-microbial in soap products which is another endocrine disruptor, especially affecting the thyroid and reproductive organs.

Sodium laureth sulfate (SLS) is the ingredient that causes foaming in soaps. The scary truth behind SLS is that it can mix with other chemicals causing severe kidney and respiratory issues, as well as hormone disruptions. Hormone disruptors interfere with the body's chemical messaging by blocking or mimicking natural hormonal actions. The more you dig into ingredient labels of common household cleaning and personal care products, the longer the toxic list will be. Ironically, basic soap and water clean just as effectively as their health damaging counterparts.

Antiperspirants contain aluminum. Anti-perspirant means "no sweat" and blocking your sweat glands with aluminum is how this is achieved. Keep in mind that your sweat glands are meant as an exit for waste. Usage of antiperspirants is strongly linked to breast cancer. The correlation between antiperspirants and breast cancer is higher among women because women generally shave their armpits, thus opening the pores to absorbing more of these chemicals then a man's hairy armpit would.

Much like foods, our environment has become so tainted with chemicals that it can seem impossible to avoid them. It is impossible to completely avoid all these substances because they are present in the air and water, as well as building materials and fabrics. The good news is that we can make a significant impact on our health and our levels of exposure by making clean pure choices where possible. Buddha Belly has included some of our favorite DIY recipes for some common body and cleaning products. There are many more natural options than what is in this chapter, but we have share some of the most important substitutions which happen to be very effective and easy to make.

Pure body products

DEODORANT
1/4 cup coconut oil melted
1/4 cup cornstarch
1/4 cup baking soda
10 drops of desires essential oil

*Mix all ingredients until a paste forms. Pour the paste into desired jar or tin and refrigerate for an hour to solidify. Mixture will vary in consistently depending on temperature so we recommend keeping in a sealed container for warm climates and situations.

FACE WASH
3 tablespoons coconut oil, melted
3 tablespoons baking soda
5 drops of desired essential oil

*Combine all ingredients and keep in small container. If the mixture gets too solid just rub between palms until it forms a cream consistently and rinse after use. Larger batches can be made after you gauge how much will be used before ingredients will expire.

SWEET BODY SCRUB
1 cup coconut oil
1/2 cup brown sugar
3 tablespoons ground cinnamon

*Melt coconut oil, but do not heat it up. Next, add other two ingredients and mix to form a sandy consistency. Store in a jar and use as an exfoliant. Rinse when done.

BODY WHIPPED CREAM
1 cup solid coconut oil
20 drops chosen essential oil

*Add solid coconut oil and essential oil to a bowl and mix on medium high for 6-7 minutes until a thick whip forms. Store in closed container and use in place of body lotions.

MINERALIZING TOOTHPASTE
3 tablespoons coconut oil
3 tablespoons pink Himalayan sea salt
3 tablespoons baking soda
10 drops peppermint essential oil

* Melt coconut oil and mix in other ingredients. Keep mixture in a jar and spoon out for each use.

BUG REPELLENT
4 ounces witch hazel
4 ounces distilled water
25 drops tea tree oil
25 drops eucalyptus oil

* Mix all ingredients and put in a glass spray bottle, or divide between multiple small bottles.

Home products

GLASS CLEANER
1/4 cup distilled water
1/4 cup vinegar
5 drops chosen essential oil

* Mix all ingredients together and keep in a glass jar or glass spray bottle. Avoid plastic containers and store labeled in fridge.

SURFACE GRIME CLEANER
1/2 cup vegetable oil
1 cup baking soda

* Mix the two ingredients together to form a paste and scrub into grimy areas with a sponge. Rinse when finished.

LAUNDRY DETERGENT
2 pounds baking soda
12 oz. Epsom salts
2 pounds washing soda
1 (4oz) bar castle soap
1.5 containers of Oxyclean baby

*Mix all ingredients and store in glass container. Use about 2 tablespoons per large load. Adjust if necessary.

TOILET BOWL DISCS
1.5 cups baking soda
1/2 cup lemon juice
25 drops lemon essential oil

*Mix all ingredients together and divide into cupcake tins. Let sit until dry. Once dry, store in bags and use one in the back of toilet (in the tank) when needed.

FLOOR CLEANER
1 cup white vinegar
1 tablespoon liquid castile soap
1 cup baking soda
10 drops essential oil
2 gallons tap water

*Mix all ingredients into a mop bucket, stir until baking soda dissolve. Warm water will help this process. Use on floors and discard when finished.

Ten

PROBIOTICS AND SUPER HEALING FOODS

Think of the little microorganisms in your body like little fish in a fish tank. I am not an expert on fish or fish tanks but I feel confident enough to use this analogy. A fish tank is its own little ecosystem. If you fill it with the right variety of fish, clean it regularly and plant the right plants, the water should stay clean enough to provide the oxygen necessary for the fish's survival. With that said, the fish still need to eat, so you must feed them accordingly. Failing to do this will starve the fish to death and throw off the balance of the tank. Assuming the tank has a variety of fish, such as bottom feeders who clean the muck off the bottom of the tank, you can see why the loss of this life would interfere with the function of the tank. On top of this, you lose fish every day to old age.

Your body is like the fish tank with the bacteria in your gut and throughout your body being the fish. Like the fish, the bacteria need to eat to be strong. If they are not fed, then they become weak and will not optimally contribute to the ecosystem of the tank. If fish are lost, new ones also need to be added to the tank in order to maintain balance. So, if your body is like the tank and your microbiome is the fish, then what is the fish food?

Prebiotics (not to be confused with probiotics) are what feed the microbiome. They are your fish food. Prebiotics are plant fibers that the body can't digest. It instead saves these nutrients for the gut bacteria to feed on. Prebiotics are found in whole foods such as fruits, vegetables, garlic, onions, and other plant based foods. Consuming an adequate amount of healthy plant foods is very essential to maintaining the health of your gut bacteria. This is easily done following the Buddha belly eating plan.

Back to probiotics, or your "fish." Probiotics need to be replenished frequently. How we go about doing that is by taking an oral supplement. While this is part of the Buddha Belly protocol, relying on supplement form alone isn't necessarily enough. Probiotics are very sensitive and often can be killed off in the stomach acid, or by heat, before ever reaching their destination in the gut. Another challenge to probiotics in supplemental form is that scientists still don't know exactly which bacteria benefit which people. Because there are so many strains and the need for different strains differ from person to person, it is currently impossible to make a supplement that will benefit all persons. This is why Buddha Belly recommends a multi strain that contains L. Bifidus and L. acidophilus since these are the strains known to support digestive health in general. Also, look for enteric coated capsules which have a strong coating to withstand stomach acid, as well as a supplement that is non-GMO and preferably raw. Avoid the brands that contain sugar in their probiotics. This should be listed in the ingredients list.

Aside from using supplemental forms of probiotics, we can benefit from consuming probiotics in the form of natural foods. Foods that have been fermented to some degree will contain natural probiotics. Buddha Belly advocates natural sources whenever possible. Nature knows more about what our bodies need then science ever will and focusing on natural sources of probiotics in foods is an efficient way to let nature suggest the adequate combination of bacteria. Kefir, kombucha, yogurt, sauerkraut, aged cheeses, sourdough, beer, wine and vinegar are all natural sources of probiotics. Since Buddha Belly excludes dairy, alcohol and wheat during the first phase, we have emphasized alternative food sources of probiotics and have included recipes for these. This will allow you to incorporate them into your health regimen and maximize the opportunity to strengthen your microbiome.

KEFIR

Kefir is a yogurt-like drink, originally made by adding culture "grains" to milk. These cultures are made of yeast and lactic acid. The cultures feed on the milk sugars causing them to ferment. The process takes about 24 hours. When making dairy kefir, raw, organic milk should be used. Even those with a lactose intolerance may be able to tolerate milk in raw form, especially once fermented. If you really don't do well with cow's milk, raw goat's milk has smaller lactose molecules and is even easier on digestion. Although milk kefir is superior to any other form of kefir, during the first phase of Buddha Belly, we recommend coconut milk kefir. Although it doesn't possess the strength of milk kefir, it will provide many of the same benefits while you are healing your gut enough to reintroduce raw dairy products.

Recipe (Coconut Milk):
2 tablespoons kefir grains
2 cups canned organic coconut milk
2 cups regular unsweetened organic coconut milk
Glass jar
Mesh cloth

* Combine coconut milk in the glass jar and add the kefir grains. Cover with mesh using a rubber band and set in a warm place for 24 hours. After 12 hours, stir the mixture well. After the 24hr fermentation period, strain the kefir through a fine strainer and keep in the fridge for up to a week. Save the grains in a glass jar in the fridge for later use. Mixture will smell like yeast. You can add vanilla for flavor or a small amount of maple syrup but we recommend adding this individually before consumption since sugar can negatively impact the grains.

KOMBUCHA

Kombucha is a drink made from tea and using a yeast bacteria Scobey, or starter. The starter feeds off the sugar in the sweet tea causing fermentation. Kombucha isn't as potent in beneficial bacteria as kefir, but still provides health benefits. The yeast causes an almost carbonated effect. Kombucha can be made from any kind of tea, but we recommend an organic tea, free of chemicals. Black varieties are commonly used to make kombucha. Small amounts of kombucha are allowed in all phases of the Buddha Belly protocol.

Recipe:
15 cups filtered water
1 cup sugar
10 teaspoons lose leaf tea or 10 tea bags
2 tablespoons apple cider vinegar with the mother
Half gallon Mason jar
Coffee filter

*Start by bringing the water to a boil in a pot. Add in the tea and let steep for 10 minutes. Stir in sugar until it dissolves, then filter the tea and pour into Mason jar. Add the vinegar and the Scobey to the jar and cover the top using the coffee filter and securing with a rubber band. Let sit in a warm dark place for 5 to 30 days. Once you smell a sour odor, you know the process is working and you can taste test it to reach your desired level of fermentation. Once the kombucha is where you would like it, transfer it to separate bottles and leave bottles at room temperature for a few days to add extra carbonation. The remaining Scobey should be divided into two parts, the main mother Scobey (your starter) and the "baby" that grew off of it. Keep these in glass jars submerged in a little kombucha liquid, in your fridge, covered for later use.

Buddha Belly puts a strong emphasis on the consumption of fermented foods. Kefir is a powerhouse of probiotics and kombucha is an enjoyable alternative to sodas and juices, while adding healthy bacteria. Aside from these two drinks, you can get probiotics from fermented foods like sauerkraut, kimchee and pickles. We recommend making your own or purchasing raw organic varieties that don't use artificial chemicals, sugar and dyes. An easy way to add more good bacteria to your gut is by consuming organic apple cider vinegar with the mother. The "mother" is the active culture present in vinegar that is responsible for its probiotic content. Apple cider vinegar can be used for everything from stomach aches to cleaning. I even used it to remove a wart my son had! If it is too strong for you to shoot straight, you can dilute it with some water. I recommend two tablespoons first thing in the morning.

What's all the hype about bone broth?

Bone broth is a substance resulting from cooking the marrow and cartilage out of meat, bones and ligaments. At a cool temperature, it is like a jelly and when heated turns to liquid. Bone broth was originally the way people made soups and stews and maximized all of the animals that they killed for nutrition purposes. Nowadays you can buy different stock from chicken to beef, but it is mainly flavored with MSG (a very unhealthy salt additive), other fillers, and artificial flavors.

Real, wholesome bone broth can easily be made at home and is an excellent complement to the Buddha Belly regimen.

Bone broth is high in collagen which helps the elasticity of the skin. Lack of elasticity in our skin is what contributes to sag, wrinkles and cellulite. Bone broth is also high in glucosamine which not only helps joint pain and function, but also heal a leaky gut. As stated before, leaky gut is a condition where there are holes present in the lining of the intestines and in order to help these heal, we need to cultivate a healthy bacterial presence and feed the body nutrients for proper tissue repair. Hence, glucosamine, which can also be taken in the form of a supplement, but like all things, the natural form is recommended as an easier and gentler way to get this hearty nutrient.

Bone broth is rich in many vitamins and minerals, phosphorus, calcium and magnesium which are present in the bones and marrow and are cooked out into a liquid form that surpasses any supplement. They contribute to joint and bone health, as well as an increased immune system. These are just some of the reasons why bone broth is being hailed as a "superfood." The benefits of it are pretty super, and unlike supplemental l-glutamine, anyone can consume it, pregnant or nursing women, etc. It is very important to remember to acquire the bones through a healthy source. Organic grass -fed or wild animal bones are best. Anything the animal comes in contact with through diet and environment will be found inside their tissues, so unless you want to drink concentrated amounts of chemicals and junk with your broth, then make sure the source is clean. Although bone broth can be made in different ways, we have included a tried and true version that we have found to have the best results.

BONE BROTH IN THE SLOW COOKER

Bones from grass finished chicken or beef (enough to fit in your slow cooker)

2 tablespoons organic apple cider vinegar

1/2 cup onion

2 cloves organic garlic

1 tablespoon pink Himalayan sea salt (optional)

* (optional) Roast bones in oven at 400 degrees for 30 minutes if raw

Place bones in crock pot and add enough water just to cover. Cook on low for 12 hours. Add remaining ingredients and cook for another 12 hours. Strain and place in fridge. When mixture cools, remove fat off top and use or freeze within 3 days.

Eleven

EATING AND HEALING IN 3 PHASES

B y this point in your journey through this book, I hope you feel enlightened to new information and motivated to do things differently than you have thus far. This is the exciting part of the process! Making strict dietary changes can be very overwhelming so during this time there are a few things to keep in mind.

Once the sugar is out, your ability to adhere to a new way of eating will become so much easier.

Sugar is said to be eight. times as addictive as cocaine and anyone with a sweet tooth can see why. It is in the majority of processed foods keeping your body suffering and addicted. By following the elimination portion, you will rid your body of the intense cravings through stabilizing blood sugars and removing chemicalized forms of sugar from your body.

When all else fails, meditate.

If stress is getting the better part of you, stop what you're doing and practice breathing and calming your mind. Schedule this time every day, more than once if necessary.

Just keep moving.

Walk. Dance. Do yoga. Whatever you do, just don't stop moving within a healthy degree. This will keep your mood strong and distract you from thoughts about food while detoxing.

You are not dieting!

Nurturing your body into a state of health and well-being is like drinking orange juice when you are sick. It is a way to heal yourself so that you get back to great.

Enjoy the accomplishments.

Don't stress on the distance in front of you. Enjoy the present moment. You own <u>this</u> moment and that's all you need to focus on.

Pretty soon you'll wake up and wonder why you ever thought you couldn't do this.

That day is just around the corner.

Rather than focus on what not to eat, let's start with what foods to eat!

FOODS TO FOCUS ON:

Vegetables: The presence of veggies is the one commonality in the majority of "diets" and so it should be. Vegetables, especially raw greens, will provide you immense fiber and nutrition, as well as bulk to fill up your belly, leaving you satisfied and full of energy after meals.

Wild, grass fed animal products: Organic animals that have lived on their natural diet are the best form of nutrition for healing your gut. A majority of the meat, eggs and dairy in the US is factory farmed. These animals are inoculated with numerous antibiotics and hormones. They are also kept in confined spaces and fed GMO corn and soy based foods that their bodies were never intended to consume. Because of this, their meat and products are chemically tainted, high in omega 6 fats, and carry a much greater risk of salmonella. Buddha belly does not advocate basing your meals around animal products, however we have found a moderate amount to be necessary in the process of gut healing because of the need for collagen in tissue repair. Look for grass finished, organic meats and eggs. Wild game is even better.

Organic fruits: Eating organic fruits in moderation will help fuel your carbohydrate intake as well as provide vitamins and minerals. Do not consume fruit in the form of juice as this is lacking fiber and will raise blood sugars too fast.

Healthy fats: Balanced amounts of healthy fats such as olive oil, coconut oil and avocado oil are a welcomed addition to Buddha belly's focus plan. These fats will provide you with energy as well as nutrition while soothing your gut.

Nuts and seeds: With the exception of peanuts, which are actually a legume, nuts and seeds consumed in moderate amounts will benefit your healing process, much like healthy oils, by providing fats and essential nutrients.

Quinoa, although similar to a grain, is actually a seed and small amounts are fine. Those with certain conditions such as diverticulitis should avoid nuts but most others will be fine with small amounts intermixed in their diet.

Potatoes: Small amounts of potatoes will provide a nutritious source of carbohydrates and fiber. We advocate sweet potatoes over white varieties due to their lower glycemic index and nutrient density. For those with insulin sensitivity, be mindful not to over consume potatoes. Instead rely more on vegetables and quinoa for your carbohydrates.

Recommended supplements for the first 30 days: multi-strain, quality probiotic (specified in chapter 10), vitamin D, magnesium, digestive enzyme for main meals to aid in digestion, quality grass fed collagen protein to assist in intestinal tissue repair and include in breakfast smoothie, bone broth (consumed at least 3 times a week and up to 7 times weekly).

*As with everything Buddha Belly preaches, listen to your body. If you have consistent negative reactions to any of these suggested foods, avoid them for the first 30 days and then try them again during the reintroduction phase.

Phase I: The first 30 days

The purpose of the first 30 days is to remove foods from the diet that are common allergens and gut irritants, as well as processed non-foods. One reason for this is to allow the gut to begin to heal while focusing on re-colonizing the probiotic bacteria. The other purpose of the first 30 days is to detox the body from addictive substances such as refined sugars, processed foods and alcohol so that a nurturing diet becomes easier.

Depending on where your current dietary habits are at, and what level of toxin buildup exists in your body, you may experience a variety of symptoms. It is common when detoxing to experience cold like symptoms as well as intestinal changes. If you experience intestinal changes that remain after a couple days or are associated to specific foods, consider that it could be that food triggering an unpleasant response and remove it for the time being. Headaches are also common, as are mood swings. These are especially present in those coming off of refined sugars and caffeine. Herbal teas and the use of essential oils can help lessen the discomfort of these withdrawal symptoms.

During this period, physical activity is important and can alleviate discomforts and redirect energy. It is important to remember to listen to your body and not overdo it. Even basic walking is a daily practice that can be incorporated into your day and extended as your body becomes more capable. Adequate rest will allow your body to rejuvenate and rebuild, which is the point of this month. There will be no cookie cutter experience for everyone as everybody is different. It is your job to listen to yours and nurture it accordingly.

HABITS FOR THE FIRST **30** DAYS

Include:

Probiotic - Quality probiotic daily

Breakfast - Drink your breakfast (healthy smoothie recipe including grass fed collagen protein)

Snacks - Superfood Snacks (2-3 a day, recipes in back)

Vegetables - Fill half your plate with veggies for both lunch and dinner (focus on mostly raw greens)

Rest - Let your digestion rest for 12 hours each night (ex: 7pm-7am)

Fermentation - Fermented food or beverage daily (1-3 servings)

Eliminate:

Processed foods and beverages- Almost anything that requires an ingredient label is a processed food. Processed foods have a high concentration of chemicals, preservatives, refined sugars and unhealthy fats. Eliminating these foods is crucial to healing your gut.

Dairy products- Most dairy comes from cows that are fed growth hormones and excessive antibiotics. On top of this, the pasteurization process renders the lactose hard to digest and lacking nutrients. Avoid all dairy for the first 30 days. After this point, you can experiment with raw organic and fermented dairy.

Wheat, flours, gluten- Gluten is very hard on the digestion. Many of the varieties of wheat are genetically modified or have come in contact with GMOs. You will likely see substantial improvement in your symptoms by eliminating gluten.

Refined sugars- Cane sugars, sugar syrups and flavorings are all forms of refined sugars. Eliminating processed foods and avoiding adding table sugar to foods, will help eliminate their consumption. If you desire some sugar (provided you don't have insulin issues) use a small amount of real maple syrup or raw honey. Buddha belly has provided some yummy sweet options in the back, recipe portion of this book.

Grains- With the exception of small amounts of quinoa which is actually a seed, we have eliminated grains during the first phase because whole, healthy grains also come with the downside of being high in anti-nutrients or phytates. The phytate in grains is reduced when soaked, sprouted or cooked but the high carbohydrate content that does feed good bacteria also feeds the bad. Until your gut microbes are balanced, it is best to keep grains out. After the first phase, occasional small amounts of whole grains may be consumed if soaked and prepared properly.

Peanuts, beans and legumes- A lot of people have a hard time tolerating the gastrointestinal effects of beans and legumes. Along with their susceptibility to carry molds, beans are high in anti-nutrients and can be very hard on the digestive system. During the healing process, it is important to keep these out of your diet until the gut feels healed enough to experiment with them in small amounts.

Corn- Corn, and the products made from it, should be strictly avoided during the initial phase. Corn can be just as hard if not harder on the gut then gluten, and much of it is genetically modified. After the first phase, you can experiment with small amounts of organic, non-GMO varieties. Avoid all products made from corn such as cornmeal, corn syrup, cornstarch and corn oil.

Soy- Most soy in the U.S. is also genetically modified. On top of that, soy can disrupt healthy hormonal function. It is especially detrimental for those with a thyroid disorder. Soy should be avoided in all forms; edamame, soy sauce, soy lecithin and soy milk. Soy can come in a multitude of forms and names so eliminating processed foods will make it easier to avoid. For those who do not suffer with an adrenal or thyroid disorder, small, occasional amounts of organic, fermented soy may be experimented with after the first 60 days but shouldn't be used as a main source of protein.

Caffeine- Caffeine is very hard on adrenal function and sometimes on blood sugars. We recommend eliminating or reducing your intake of caffeine in general, especially through the initial healing phase. If your body reacts well to coffee, try to stick to one cup per day of organic coffee or decaf. Small amounts of organic green tea can provide a nutritious, less acidic alternative while detoxing.

Alcohol- Alcohol suppresses the immune system and slows the body's metabolic rate (fat burning). Many forms of beers and beverages are also made with high fructose corn syrups and chemicals, as well as being high in gluten. Alcohol also disrupts quality, healing sleep. In moderation, healthy alcohol options can have a place in your life after the first 30 days. During the reintroduction phase we will discuss how to choose clean drink options without back peddling on your gut's progress.

Phase 2: Reintroduction (30 days)

After the first 30 days, you can start reintroducing small amounts of certain whole foods to your gut. If you have a severe case of leaky gut and auto immune issues, you may want to extend the first phase longer than 30 days. The foods to experiment with during this phase are raw organic dairy, organic non-GMO corn, whole gluten free grains (soaked and sprouted), and small amounts of clean alcoholic beverages. Due to their negative effects on gut healing, addiction level and/or lack of nutrients, we recommend leaving refined sugars, processed foods, gluten, caffeine and soy out of your diet still at this point.

Wait at least 72 hours between food introductions and only add one at a time. Intolerant reactions can wait a day or two before showing up so in order to eliminate confusion, focus on one at a time.

When experimenting with the reintroduction of foods during this phase it is important to journal when you add something back. This will allow you to be aware of which foods your body doesn't respond well to. If you have a negative reaction to a particular food or substance, that is a good indication that that food or substance has damaged, and possibly still will damage, your gut. You will be able to use this information to make choices in the future regarding what you consume and how often.

Alcohol should be reintroduced in the same way as foods, not within a 72hr period of any other reintroduced food. You should also choose varieties that are clean such as organic red wine and clean (unsweetened) clear liquor, such as vodka. Craft beers may be tried after this month if your body responds well to wheat.

Phase 3: Developing a Buddha belly way of life

After putting in a strict and progressive 60 days you will have likely noticed some amazing things about your body, as well as your thoughts and feelings. Depending on how severe your issues were when starting this, your body may continue to improve. For others, you will want to maintain the YOU that you have nurtured into being. Here are a few tips:

- Continue to build your meals around vegetables, making this center stage
- Choose organic, properly sourced and fed animal products, fruits and veggies.
- Keep GMO's and processed foods out of your diet as much as possible, along with unhealthy fats. Refined sugar is especially addictive and can be easily substituted with natural sweeteners like raw honey and real maple syrup.

- Make probiotic rich, fermented foods a consistent part of your diet.
- Limit your intake of whole grains, corn and beans, and when consuming them, prepare them properly by soaking and sprouting prior to cooking.
- Choose raw, unpasteurized, organic dairy products.
- Remember what foods interfere with your body and your gut's homeostasis, and if you must consume these foods, save them for a rare occasion.
- Never quit moving, meditating and loving yourself!

A "baby step" approach

Buddha belly was written to share the culmination of information that has come to be at this place in time, along with over a decade of my personal education and experiences. Combining holistic health along with experiences of many contributing individuals, it was my intention to write a book that consisted of all this information in hopes that it would touch a lot of people. With that said, there are people, including those I have worked with, who may feel overwhelmed to tackle Buddha belly's full 60day process at once. Because of this, Buddha Belly has included a "baby step" approach so that everyone can use this information to start progressing their health and defying the current rate of disease. In the long run, you will all reach the finish line.

You can still follow the focus portion of the main protocol. Drinking your breakfast in the form of a healthy smoothie, consuming large amounts of mainly raw veggies with your large meals, and adding the listed supplements will naturally add nutrition as well as gut healing benefits.

FIRST 30 DAYS:

For the initial phase of the baby steps process we have chosen to eliminate the substances that are consistently hard on the body.

- Gluten
- Corn
- Artificial sweeteners

For this period you will want to avoid anything with wheat or any form of gluten present in it, all corn products and any artificial sugars.

Practice the mind, body, soul suggestions listed in the book. Relax, get adequate sleep and focus on positive thoughts and affirmations.

DAYS 31-60

At this time, you should have already noticed improvements by removing gluten, corn and artificial sweeteners. The next step is insuring that your diet consists of all whole foods. Pulling the foods listed below out of your diet will help achieve this.

- Soy
- Refined sugars
- Unhealthy fats

- Processed foods
- Alcohol

By the end of this phase you should see substantial improvements in your body and your health. Your cravings should start to become mild and easily satisfied in healthier ways.

Days 61-90

At this point in the baby steps approach your body is ready to pull some commonly irritating and allergenic foods. Below we have given you a list of the recommended foods to remove for the next 30 days, in order to allow more intense healing of the gut.

- Grains (except quinoa)
- Dairy
- Beans, legumes and peanuts
- Caffeine

By the end of this phase your gut should be significantly improved and you will be ready to experiment with reintroduction.

Reintroduction days 91-120

Follow the reintroduction and maintenance approach on previous pages

Twelve

WRAP UP AND RECIPES

*A*long my own health journey and throughout the course of writing Buddha Belly, I have been blessed to meet so many people who have contributed their own experiences with gut health. I thought it only fitting to include a couple of their stories along with my own before digging into the recipes!

"In July of 2010, I was diagnosed with Chron's disease. I had suffered for 4 years and saw 3 different Gastroenterologist's before receiving my diagnosis. My disease had progressed long enough that I was immediately placed on steroids and immunosuppressant's. After a few months, and continued pain and weight loss, it was obvious they were not working and surgery was the only option. Only 7 months after my diagnosis, I went in for surgery. They removed half of my colon and some of my small intestines, totaling about 16 inches. I was in the hospital for a week and came home weighing 88 pounds (my ideal weight is about 114).

My whole food journey did not start until about a year and a half later, when after having my first child and having a difficult delivery, I needed antibiotics. This threw my system into a tailspin. I spent the first two years of my daughter's life in the bathroom and in a lot of pain. It was a very depressing time. Tired of going the conventional route and seeing no change, I started searching on my own for answers. I went and saw a naturopath for the first time in my life. She diagnosed me with a leaky gut, something I had never heard of before. The first thing I did was completely change my diet. I ate roasted chicken thighs, cooked sweet potatoes and carrots, homemade bone broth and gelatin gummies for two months. I took large quantities of probiotics and drank the liquid from fermented vegetables. In the next two months, I was gaining weight, my bathroom trips were becoming less and less, my pain was reducing and I was finding hope again. Now, two years later, I have been able to maintain my weight, stay off prescription medications and even had a second baby without any issues. My diet is ever changing as my nutritional needs change, but the one constant is that I continue to eat a whole foods diet without gluten, soy, red meat or dairy. I hope my story is a testament that with the right foods and the proper environment, our body has the ability to heal itself."

~ Kristina (Seattle Wa)

I was always very athletic in my early years, but dealt with injuries and medical issues starting in my twenties. At the age of 43, I suffered a stroke which left me paralyzed in different sections of my body and an extreme inability to move. I have been on multiple medications for many different issues since then. Weight gain, asthma and skin conditions are just a few of the conditions I have been challenged with and that doctors have been working to "treat" all these years. I started the Buddha Belly Baby Steps program by taking out artificial sweeteners and gluten, things that none of my doctors had ever suggested. It taught me a new way to eat. Almost immediately I noticed a difference in my ability to breath and in a short time my skin cleared up. I no longer need medications for either of these conditions. I also have more energy and can walk further . . . and have lost 47 pounds! I truly appreciate what this book has done for me.

~ Rob (Spokane Wa)

Like these individuals, I have experienced my own wellness challenges throughout my life. What I discovered along my journey while writing and living Buddha Belly, was something more complex than just an improved physical state. Physically, I was able to return to my pre-baby weight while breastfeeding which is something that has always been very difficult for me. I also experienced less joint and muscle pains, improved digestion, loss of a sugar addiction and no seasonal allergies for the first time in 10 years. These

improvements were exciting and affirming, but the most powerful changes for me were in my mind. Becoming aware of my self-perception and motivating myself with a nurturing love has brought so much more peace into my life. Until this point I had thought that a chronic state of stress was normal. I never could have imagined ditching the little voice that would constantly break me down. I have not mastered these areas and to be 100 percent honest, I re-read the chapters on stress and self-appreciation frequently. I don't do this out of vanity. I read through these chapters when I feel myself forgetting to live the way I preach to others. It is much easier to show love or encourage another to love themselves then it is to love yourself. Doing this reminds me to show myself the love, grace and patience that I desire for everyone else. I am grateful for all the experiences that have brought me right where I am today, truly healthy.
Brittney Prendergast

FOCUS FOODS LIST

*INCLUDING BUT NOT LIMITED TO

GREENS
alfalfa sprouts, arugula, asparagus, basil, bean sprouts, bok choy, broccoli, butter lettuce, cabbage, celery, cucumber, collard greens, dandelion greens, fennel, green beans, kale, kelp, leafy greens, leeks, lemon grass, lettuce, mustard greens, parsley, spinach, watercress, Zucchini

COLORED VEGGIES
bell pepper, cauliflower, cherry tomatoes, chili peppers, eggplant, garlic, ginger, green peppers, jalapeno, mushrooms, okra, onions, red bell pepper, tomatillo, tomatoes, water chestnuts,

STARCHES AND GLUTEN FREE GRAINS
banana squash, beets, butternut squash, carrots, potatoes, pumpkins, squash, sweet potatoes, quinoa

HEALTHY FATS
avocado, avocado oil, coconut oil, ghee, grass fed butter, olives, olive oil, sesame oil

NUTS AND SEEDS
almonds, brazil nuts, chia seeds, hazelnuts, macadamia nuts, pecans, pistachio, sesames, sunflower seeds, walnuts

ANIMAL PROTEINS
eggs, meats and seafood *preferably Organic, grass finished, wild caught and wild game

FERMENTED FOODS
kefir, kimchi, kombucha, miso, pickles, sauerkraut, vinegar

"Loving your body with food"

Buddha Belly was written for the purpose of facilitating health through mind, body and soul. The main component of physical health is the health of your microbiome or "gut". Through Buddha Belly's elimination phase, focusing on life giving foods is essential. A diet high in fresh, organic vegetables and some fruits will keep the PH of the body in a more alkaline state, making it an undesirable environment for disease. Complementing fresh produce with clean, morally and healthily raised protein will nourish your body in a new way. Eating in a nurturing way is not only healing for the body and the gut, but with the right recipes is can be a beautiful and satisfying experience. We have included some of our favorite Buddha Belly approved recipes that are excellent for all phases of your health journey.

   * For more Gut wellness, recipes, motivation or information on becoming a certified Holistic Coach, go to www.holisticwellnesscoaches.com

Recipes

Smoothie love

CLEAN GREEN
1 cup cucumber
4oz purified water
2 handfuls spinach
1/2 small lemon (whole)
4 ice cubes

* Start with the water and then add cucumber and lemon. Blend well. Next add spinach and blend again until pureed. Lastly add ice cubes and blend to your desired consistency.

CHOCOLATE CHIA SUPERFOOD
6oz almond milk
1.5 cups chopped kale
1 small frozen banana
2Tbs chia seeds
2Tbs cocoa powder

*Start by combining milk, kale and chia seeds in blender. Blend until kale is broken down well. Next add remaining ingredients and blend to desired consistency

Smoothie Love

TROPICOLADA
1/4 cup coconut water
4oz canned coconut milk
1/2 cup frozen pineapple chunks
1/4 cup unsweetened, flaked coconut
1 tsp vanilla extract
4 ice cubes

*Combine all ingredients except ice cubes to a pureed consistency Lastly add ice cubes and blend well.

PROTEIN BERRY BLISS
6oz almond milk
1 large handful spinach
2 scoops grass fed collagen protein
1/2 cup frozen organic mixed berries

*Combine almond milk and spinach and blend to break down greens. Add remaining ingredients and blend well.

Smoothie Love

SPICY AFTER PARTY
1/4 cup purified water
1/4 cup lime juice
1 red bell pepper
1/2 cup chopped celery
2 cups chopped romaine
1 tsp cayenne
1 tsp Himalayan sea salt
5 ice cubes

*Combine water, lime juice and romaine and blend well. Add all remaining ingredients except ice and blend. Add ice and blend to desired consistency

ZESTY ITALIAN
4oz clamato juice
2 Roma tomatoes
1/2 cup cucumber
1 tsp Italian herbs
1Tbs olive oil
1 tsp black pepper
5 ice cubes

*Blend all ingredients except ice until well pureed. Add ice and blend to desired consistency.

Smoothie Love

VERY HUCKLEBERRY HEALTHY
6oz unsweetened almond milk
1/2 small avocado
1 cup chopped kale
1/2 cup frozen huckleberries

* Combine first three ingredients and blend well. Add huckleberries and blend to desired consistency

TROPI-KALE PROTEIN SMOOTHIE
4oz unsweetened almond milk
4oz coconut water
1/2 small avocado
1.5 cups chopped kale
1 serving grass fed collagen protein
1 cup frozen mango

*Combine almond milk, coconut water, avocado and kale and blend well. Add remaining ingredients and blend to desired consistency

Smoothie Love

BANANA NUT BREAKFAST
8oz unsweetened almond milk
1 frozen banana
1Tbs almond butter
1 tsp cinnamon
1Tbs maple syrup
1 tsp maple extract
3 ice cubes

* Combine all ingredients except ice and blend well. Add recommended ice or enough to achieve desired consistency

PUMPKIN PROTEIN SPICE
4oz canned coconut milk
1 frozen banana
1/2 cup pureed pumpkin
1Tbs almond butter
1 serving, grass-fed collagen protein powder

* Combine all ingredients in high powered blender and blend to desired consistency

Smoothie Love

CREAMY CHOCOLATE OMEGA
6oz unsweetened almond milk
1/2 small avocado
2Tbs chia seeds
1.5 cups chopped spinach
1/2 frozen banana
2Tbs cocoa powder
3 ice cubes

*Combine first four ingredients and blend well. Add remaining ingredients and blend to consistency

SWEET GREEN APPLES
6oz coconut water
1 small green apple
1 cup spinach
1 cup kale
1/2 small lemon (with rind)
5 ice cubes

Blend all ingredients except ice. Blend well to break down fiber. Add ice and blend to desired consistency

Smoothie Love

MANGO MACRO MIRACLE

8oz coconut water
1 cup microgreens of choice (mint, parsley etc. experiment with them all!)
2Tbs chia seeds
1/2 cup frozen mango

*Combine coconut water with greens and chia seeds and blend well. Add frozen mango and blend to consistency

RASPBELLY- BIOTIC

6oz kefir (coconut milk kefir or raw goats milk kefir)
1 cup chopped kale
1/2 cup chopped leek
1 cup frozen organic raspberries
1Tbs raw honey
1 tsp vanilla extract

* Combine kefir, kale and leek and blend well. Add frozen berries and blend to desired consistency

Full Belly Salads

Cajun Shrimp Superfood Salad (2 large servings, 4 small)

3 large handfuls kale
1 cup quinoa (uncooked)
1lb large shrimp
1 large avocado chopped
1/2 cup diced sweet onion
2 cloves garlic chopped
4 stalks celery chopped
4Tbs olive oil
2Tbs lemon juice
2 tsp cumin
1 tsp cayenne pepper
sea salt to taste

* Start by preparing the quinoa. I like to recommended using a small crock pot. Mix a 1:2 ratio of quinoa to water and let cook on low for about 1.5 hours. You can make extra in a large crock to use for other recipes. Wash and dry kale and chop into small pieces. Chop avocado, garlic, celery. Use half of the cumin and cayenne and sprinkle on shrimp. Combine olive oil and lemon juice with remaining spices including salt and set aside. Add all chopped ingredients along with shrimp and quinoa to a large bowl and toss with dressing mixture.

Full Belly Salads

BLACKBERRIES AND TURKEY SALAD WITH BLACKBERRY VINAIGRETTE (2 LARGE SERVINGS, 4 SMALL)

6 cups mixed greens
3/4 cup chopped avocado
1 cup cooked turkey breast chopped
1/2 cup red onion thinly sliced
1/4 cup slivered almonds
3/4 cup blackberries whole

BLACKBERRY VINAIGRETTE

2Tbs olive oil
2Tbs white wine vinegar
1Tbs raw honey
1/2 cup blackberries
1 tsp sea salt

* Chop all ingredients, toss together lightly and set aside in a large bowl. Mix dressing in blender, bullet or food processor and puree well. Toss dressing into salad. You can choose to leave the almonds and whole blackberries out until the end allowing you to garnish them on top of salad, making for a much more esthetically appealing plate.

Full Belly Salads

SMOKED SALMON COBB WITH COCONUT RANCH (2 LARGE SERVINGS OR 4 SMALL)

6 cups romaine chopped
1 cup cherry tomatoes sliced in half
1/2 red onion sliced into fine pieces
4 hardboiled eggs
6oz smoked salmon cut into bite sized pieces
1 small avocado cut into chunks

Dressing:
1/2 tsp black pepper
1/2 tsp chives
1/2 tsp sea salt
3/4 tsp onion powder
3/4 tsp garlic powder
1Tbs white wine vinegar
1/2 tsp parsley
1/2 tsp oregano
1 can of coconut milk (cream only)

*Slice romaine, tomatoes and onion and toss together. Slice hard boiled eggs and add to top of salad along with salmon and avocado. Mix dressing using some of the coconut liquid if necessary until you reach desired consistency Drizzle over entire salad or individual portions.

Full Belly Salads

Pineapple chicken teriyaki salad

6 cups chopped romaine
2/3 cup chunked pineapple (in 100% juice)
1/2 red onion sliced
1 orange bell pepper, sliced into strips
2 cups chicken breast cubed

Dressing:
1.5 Tbs coconut aminos
2.5 Tbs extra virgin olive oil
2 tsp honey
1 Tbs apple cider vinegar
1/2 clove garlic diced fine
1/8 tsp ginger
sea salt to taste

* Prepare chicken breast and set aside. Chop romaine, pepper and onion and toss together in a large bowl. Add chicken and pineapple. In a separate container, mix dressing and pour over salad. Salt to taste

Full Belly Salads

Protein packed potato salad

6 medium russet potatoes

1/2 purple onion diced

3 stalks celery chopped

3 hardboiled eggs

2 cups cubed chicken breast

1 large head romaine lettuce

4Tbs olive oil

1Tbs paprika

3 tsp sea salt

2 tsp black pepper

2Tbs Italian seasoning

3Tbs white wine vinegar

2Tbs worcestershire sauce

3Tbs mustard

* Wash and cook potatoes on a baking sheet at 375 for 50 minutes. Let cool completely and dice into chunks. Set aside. Chop onion, celery, eggs, chicken and romaine and toss together in a large bowl. Drizzle potatoes with half the olive oil and all of the spices. Add spiced potatoes to bowl and toss. Combine remaining olive oil, mustard, vinegar and worcestershire sauce. Toss until coated evenly.

Full Belly Salads

SWEET CHICKEN DEJON SALAD
5 cups chopped romaine
1 cup chopped mustard greens
1/2 cup green onions
1 cup cooked quinoa
2 cups chicken breast cubed

dressing:
3Tbs olive oil
2Tbs Dejon mustard
2Tbs raw honey
2Tbs white wine vinegar
1 tsp sea salt
2 tsp black pepper

* Mix dressing ingredients and set aside. Chop romaine, mustard greens and onions and toss together. Add quinoa and chicken and mix well. Toss in dressing.

Nourishing Soups and Sautes

SHRIMP AND CAULIFLOWER BONE BROTH CHOWDER

1lb cocktail shrimp
1 can full fat coconut milk
16oz bone broth
1Tbs coconut oil
1 medium head cauliflower
2 stocks celery
2 tsp sea salt
1 tsp black pepper
1Tbs dill weed

* In a large fry pan, heat coconut oil. Chop celery and cauliflower and add to the pan. Saute the veggies until semi-firm. Add remaining ingredients and cook on medium for another 5-10 minutes until heated through.

Nourishing Soups and Sautes

MEXICAN CHICKEN CHILI (4 MEDIUM PORTIONS)
1lb chicken breast sliced
1(14oz) can full fat coconut milk
2 cups bone broth
1 can Mexican diced tomatoes (no sweetener)
1 (4oz) can diced green chilis
2Tbs coconut oil
1/2 large sweet onion diced
4 stocks of celery diced
2Tbs sea salt
1 tsp chili powder
2 tsp cumin

* Chop chicken breast into medium strips and set aside. Dice onion and celery. In a large frying pan, heat coconut oil on medium heat. Dice onion and celery and add to the frying pan. Saute veggies until semi softened. Add sea salt, chili powder and cumin and cook for 1 minute. Pour coconut milk and bone broth over mixture and reduce heat slightly. Lastly add cooked chicken and cook another 4 minutes, stirring frequently

Nourishing Soups and Sautes

EGG DROP QUINOA SOUP (2 SERVINGS)

1 Tbs coconut oil
4 eggs
1/2 cup chopped chives
1.5 cups cooked quinoa
1.5 cups bone broth
1/2 cup water
2 tsp basil
1 tsp black pepper
sea salt to taste

* Start by scrambling eggs in coconut oil and chopping into small pieces. Set aside. Next, heat bone broth on medium low and add green onion. Heat for 5 minutes or until desired temperature is reached. Be careful not to overheat or you will lose the benefits of the bone broth. Add quinoa and egg along with seasoning. Sea salt to taste.

This is a great soup to substitute instant noodles and processed chicken noodle.

Nourishing Soups and Sautes

FAJITA FRI (2 LARGE SERVINGS, 4 SMALL)
1 red bell pepper
1 yellow bell pepper
1 medium yellow onion sliced into strips
2 cups broccoli straws
2 cups chopped chicken breast (cooked)
2Tbs coconut oil
2Tbs coconut aminos
1 tsp cayenne pepper
1 tsp chili powder
2 tsp cumin
2 tsp lime juice
sea salt

* In a large frying pan or wok, add coconut oil and heat on medium. Chop onion and peppers and saute lightly in coconut oil along with broccoli straws. Once the veggies are cooked to a semi- firm consistency, turn the heat down to med low and add chopped chicken. Mix in remaining spices and toss to coat. Sea salt to taste.

Nourishing Soups and Sautes

SUNNY OVER SPINACH (2 LARGE SERVINGS, 4 SMALL)

6 cups spinach
2Tbs Coconut oil
1 tsp sea salt
4 free range eggs
Coconut aminos

* In a large frying pan, add coconut oil and spinach. Saute until lightly wilted but not fully cooked down. Add sea salt to top of spinach and pat down to form a "nest" or semi-flat surface. Crack eggs over top of spinach. Cover and cook on medium for approximately 3 minutes. Check eggs to determine your desired level of "done". Once the eggs are cooked to your liking, remove the pan from heat, let cool for 2 minutes, top with coconut aminos and serve. Mixture should hold together in a fritatta-like form.

Note: Meals such as this one are fast, simple and healthy. You can prepare this for breakfast, lunch or dinner and even add a side of cooked diced potatoes for those who need more calories.

Nourishing soups and sautes

BROCCOLI STEAK STIR FRY (2 LARGE PORTIONS OR 4 SMALL)
5 cups whole organic broccoli
2 cups steak cubed
2Tbs water
1Tbs olive oil
2Tbs worcestershire
1.5Tbs coconut aminos
1 tsp black pepper
sea salt to taste

* Start by cooking steak to desired tenderness. Cut the steak into cubes before or after its cooked and set aside. Add water and broccoli to a large frying pan and cook, covered on medium heat, stirring occasionally. Cool broccoli until firm but not hard. Once done, turn heat down to med-low and stir in remaining ingredients. Cook for another 5 minutes.

Hearty Meals

BASIL BALSAMIC ROASTED SALMON OVER HERBED QUINOA
2Tbs worcestershire sauce
1Tbs balsamic vinegar
1 tsp basil
1 tsp pink Himalayan sea salt
2 (4oz) wild salmon fillets

HERBED QUINOA
2 cups cooked quinoa
1 tsp basil
1 tsp onion powder
1 tsp rosemary
2 tsp sea salt (or to taste)
1 tsp black pepper
2Tbs olive oil

* Pre-heat the oven to 375. Mix the worcestershire and vinegar and pour over salmon fillets in a deep rimmed baking dish or pan. Sprinkle basil and salt over fillets and bake for 18 minutes or until done.

For the quinoa, heat oil over med heat in a frying pan and add quinoa. Heat until slightly crisp. Add remaining ingredients and cook another 2 minutes.

Serve salmon over a bed of quinoa or on the side and next to a large helping of steamed veggies or salad.

Hearty Meals

DEEP DISH PIZZA WITH QUINOA CRUST
2 cups cooked quinoa
2Tbs Italian seasoning
1Tbs sea salt
2 fresh eggs
1Tbs olive oil

*Start by preheating oven to 350. Mix all ingredients for crust in a medium bowl. Grease a 10-12 in pie pan with olive oil and press quinoa mixture down into it and against sides. Bake for 15 minutes or until golden brown.

TOPPING OPTIONS
Pizza sauce (no sweetener added)
Avocado slices
Onions
Olives
Pesto sauce
Chicken
Smoked salmon
Mushrooms

The possibilities are endless as long as they are clean so get creative and indulge in a favorite food that is healthy for your belly.

Hearty Meals

WILD TENDERLOIN AND MUSHROOMS (2 LARGE SERVINGS)

1lb of wild meat tenderloin (we use elk or venison)
2lbs of sliced mushrooms of choice
2Tbs grass fed butter
1 whole white onion
2Tbs worcestershire sauce
Sea salt to taste

* Chop mushrooms and onion into large piece and set aside. In a large frying pan add 1Tbs butter and tenderloin meat. Cook over medium heat until cooked through. Once done, remove meat and set aside. Saute mushrooms and onions in leftover meat juice. Once cooked to a semi soft consistency, add in the meat and remaining ingredients. Heat together for another 3 minutes and serve.

Hearty Meals

BBQ CHICKEN STUFFED SWEET POTATOES (4 SERVINGS)
4 medium sweet potatoes
1/2lb organic free range chicken breast diced
1/2 large white onion
1Tbs olive oil
2Tbs grassfed butter
sea salt to taste

BBQ SAUCE
6oz can of organic tomato paste
8oz organic applesauce
2Tbs balsamic vinegar
1/4 tsp black pepper
1/2 tsp onion powder
1/2 tsp garlic powder
1/2 tsp worcestershire sauce
1/2 tsp coconut aminos

* Preheat oven to 400 degrees. Wash sweet potatoes and poke with knife 3 times. Cook potatoes at 400 degrees for 20 minutes then turn the heat down to 350 for a remaining 60 minutes. Mix BBQ sauce ingredients and set aside. Cook diced chicken in a fry pan, and add 3Tbs BBQ sauce. Cook for another 2 minutes and set aside. Chop onions and saute in olive oil until softened. Add to chicken mixture. When potatoes are done, let cool slightly and cut slightly down the middle of each. Add butter and salt to potato and mash together. Top each potato with 1/4 of chicken mixture.

Hearty Meals

WILD SHEPHERD'S PIE

Filling:
2 cups chopped mushrooms
1 can Mexican diced tomatoes
1 chopped onion
3/4 cup olives diced
1/2lb ground meat (we used venison)
1/2 cup tomato paste
1Tbs chili powder
1 tsp cumin
1/2Tbs salt

Topping:
1/2 cup gluten free flour
1/2 cup almond meal
1Tbs honey
1 Egg
1/2 cup almond milk
1Tbs coconut oil
1/2 tsp salt

* For the filling, start by chopping the onions and olives while cooking in a frying pan the ground meat of choice until thoroughly cooked. Next add all the remaining ingredients except for tomato paste until sauteed down a bit. Don't let veggies get too soggy seeing as how they will continue to cook in the oven but this will help some of the moisture to

leave the veggies. Next add tomato paste and seasonings and set aside.

*Start your topping by mixing the gluten free flour and almond meal along with salt. Next add the milk, honey and coconut oil and set aside.

* To combine I used two 4x8 in loaf pans (double recipe for large family or leftovers) and split the filling between the two pans like pictured above. Next split the cornmeal topping between the two pans and spread over top. The filling won't be super thick which allows this recipe to be less heavy then commonly prepared and very balanced with protein and veggies. (still so yummy!)
Bake in a preheated oven at 375 F for aprox 17 minutes. Once done, let cool for 5 mins and serve with side salad or raw veggie of choice!

Hearty Meals

SMOKED SALMON QUINOA CAKES
2.5 cups cooked quinoa
3/4lb smoked salmon flaked or cut into small bits
4 eggs
1/2 cup onion diced
1 large clove garlic diced
2 tsp sea salt
1 tsp black pepper
2 tsp dried basil
olive oil

* Chop onion and garlic and set aside. In a large mixing bowl, beat all eggs well and add onion, garlic, salt, pepper and basil and mix well. Fold in salmon and quinoa. Heat a non-stick pan to medium and coat with olive oil. Using 1/4 measuring cup, scoop mixture and place in pan. Flatten down into a 1/2in patty and cook each side until done (aprox 3 minutes each side. Serve with a large amount of veggies or over a bed of greens.

Sweet treats and superfood snacks

FROSTED FUDGY RAW BROWNIES
2.5 cups pitted dates
3/4 cup walnuts
1/2 cup cocoa powder
1/8 tsp sea salt
1 Tbs coconut oil

FROSTING
3 Tbs coconut oil
3 Tbs maple syrup
1 tsp vanilla extract
1/2 cup cocoa powder

* In a high-grade blender or food processor add dates, walnuts cocoa powder, salt and coconut oil. Blend well until a crumply but slightly sticky consistency results. In a 8x5 loaf pan, press brownie mixture evenly and tightly. Mix frosting ingredients. If oil is solid you can melt it in a bowl by sitting the bowl in a pan of hot water.
Spread frosting mixture over brownies and place in freezer for at least 15 minutes. Cut and serve. Brownies can be stored in freezer, fridge or room temp but the frosting will change consistency depending on what temperature it is stored at.
* You can experiment with the recipe by adding raspberry flavoring, mint etc.

Sweet Treats and Superfood Snacks

MACADAMIA BUTTER BARS

BAR INGREDIENTS:
1 cup cashew butter
1/4 cup coconut oil
1/4 cup Maple syrup
1/4 cup macadamia nuts
1/3 cup unsweetened coconut
pinch of salt

WHITE CHOCOLATE TOPPING:
1Tbs coconut oil
2Tbs Honey or maple
1/4 cup coconut milk cream
1 tsp vanilla
1/4 cup unsweetened coconut

*Start by melting the coconut oil and adding this and the cashew butter to a food processor along with maple and pulse for aprox 30 seconds and then add coconut and salt and pulse for another 20 seconds. Scrape mixture into a clean bowl and stir in Macadamia nuts. Line a loaf pan with parchment paper allowing it to hang over so it can be easily removed. (I used a 5x5 glass pan for thicker bars)
Pour first part of bar mixture into pan and place in freezer.

*Topping: Melt the coconut oil and add maple and vanilla then fold in the coconut cream. To get the coconut "cream" place a can of full fat coconut milk in fridge for a few hours, take top off and skim thick cream off top. Use extra liquid in smoothies etc.

Lastly fold in 1/4 cup coconut and pour over top of bars and place in freezer for at least an hour or more.

Sweet Treats and Superfood Snacks

DARK CHOCOLATE ALMOND BARK
1/2 cup melted coconut oil
3Tbs pure maple syrup
1/2 cup cocoa powder
1/2 cup raw almonds
1 tsp pink Himalayan sea salt (optional)

* Start by melting coconut oil in a bowl set in a larger pan of hot water. Add syrup and cocoa powder and mix well. Add almonds and stir to coat.
Pour mixture into a 5x8 loaf pan and sprinkle sea salt on top. Place in freezer for 30 minutes.
Break the bark into pieces and store in a container in the freezer.

Sweet Treats and Superfood Snacks

SWEET POTATO FRIES

2 large sweet potatoes
2Tbs olive oil
sea salt to taste

* Pre-heat oven to 375
Wash and dry sweet potatoes and remove the skin. Chop into long fry slices or rounds approximately 1/4 inch thick.
Coat fries in olive oil and place large baking sheet as separated as possible
Sprinkle with sea salt and bake for 45 minutes
At the 25minute mark, remove fries and turn with spatula to prevent uneven cooking

Sweet Treats and Superfood Snacks

KALE CHIPS
One large bushel of kale
3Tbs olive oil
sea salt to taste

* Wash and dry kale really well. If need be, wash ahead of time and lay out to dry or use a paper towel.
Preheat oven to 350
Remove stem from kale and rip or tear into chip size pieces
Coat kale evenly in olive oil and spread over large baking sheet
Bake for 10 minutes and turn over with a spatula
cook for another 10 minutes or until crispy and slightly browned

* Kale chips make an easy and delicious side for any hearty meal as well as an excellent alternative to chips.

Teas

ELECTROLYTE TEA
10 tsp lose leaf tea (we recommend a fruity non-caffeinated variety)
1/2 gallon purified water
1/2gallon mason jar
2 tsp pink Himalayan sea salt
4Tbs fresh lemon juice
4Tbs raw honey (optional)

* Brew tea by steeping loose leafs in hot water for at least 10 minutes before straining and let cool.
You can cold brew it as well the night before by adding leaves to room temperature water and letting sit for 12-24 hours before straining
Once tea is brewed and warm but not hot. Add remaining ingredients, mix until dissolved and keep in mason jar in the fridge.

Teas

COCONUT SPICED CHAI
2 tsp lose leaf spiced chai tea blend
16oz purified water

* Heat the water until it's just about to boil
steep chai blend for at least 10 minutes for extra flavor
while steeping, mix creamer

SUPER COCONUT CREAMER
1 Can Organic Coconut milk
12oz of nut milk (unsweetened) I like almond:)
2Tbs of melted down LOCAL, RAW HONEY
2 tsp vanilla extract

You will firstly want to melt the honey down by putting it in
a glass container and submerging the container in a bowl of
very hot water for a few minutes (DONT use microwave!! It
kills off all those healthful bacteria and radiation doesn't taste
good:(
Next add remaining ingredients to a 20oz jar and mix well.
Shake before each use to break up coconut particles.

Teas

LEMONADE KOMBUCHA

12oz kombucha (if making yourself, we recommend a lemongrass and black tea combination)
1Tbs honey
3Tbs fresh lemon juice
4oz carbonated water

*Warm the lemon juice slightly and dissolve honey into it
Add to kombucha and mix well
top with carbonated water

*Increase recipe size for large quantities and keep in fridge

67961595R00093

Made in the USA
Lexington, KY
27 September 2017